ABOUT THE AUTHOR

Donald Norfolk is an osteopath and editor of a monthly health magazine. He is extremely aware of the need for better health education in the community and has lectured extensively on health, both in this country and abroad. He has also broadcast frequently on radio and television, and he is the author of *The Stress Factor*, also published by Hamlyn Paperbacks.

FIT FOR LIFE

Donald Norfolk

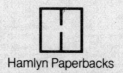

Hamlyn Paperbacks

FIT FOR LIFE

ISBN 0 600 20048 5

First published in Great Britain 1980
by Hamlyn Books
Hamlyn Paperbacks edition 1981
Copyright © 1980 by Donald Norfolk

Hamlyn Paperbacks are published by
The Hamlyn Publishing Group Ltd,
Astronaut House,
Feltham,
Middlesex, England

(Paperback Division: Hamlyn Paperbacks,
Banda House, Cambridge Grove,
Hammersmith, London W6 0LE)

Reproduced, printed and bound in Great Britain by
Cox & Wyman Ltd, Reading

CONTENTS

1

The Low-Vitality Lifestyle

Something is sadly amiss with the health of the Western world. In recent years we have recorded breathtaking advances in medical care, and yet in many ways we are less healthy than our forebears. Despite the creation of a megalithic entertainment industry, our level of discontent appears greater than ever before. With immense technological ingenuity we seem to have created a mechanically sophisticated paradise, whose only asset is that it enables us to be miserable in comfort. In lands flowing with the milk and honey of material prosperity, thousands of people lead impoverished bread-and-water lives.

Few people are really well. Most exist in a state of sub-health, inhabiting the depressing no-man's land between total fitness and frank disease. According to the most recently published *General Household Survey*, seventy per cent of Britons consider their health to be poor. Journalists have tried to dismiss this startling statistic as evidence of widespread hypochondriasis, but this is no delusion. My observation as editor of a fitness magazine, and my twenty-five years' experience as an osteopath, convince me that the health of seven out of every ten Britons is undoubtedly poor. And this is almost certainly true of every other industrialized nation.

But what is the cause of this widespread malaise? Considerable evidence has now been amassed which shows that most of this toll of sickness is self-inflicted. We are in many ways our own executioners. We are leading lives which are inimical to our physical health and psychological well-being. Over a period of many thousands of years mankind evolved as a high-activity species. Now we are attempting to lead the life of indolent sloths. Evolution has equipped us to survive the excitements and hazards of the primeval forest, not to withstand the routine passivity of urban life. So we suffer the diseases of maladaptation. The most common conditions we suffer from today – tiredness, depression, obesity, rheumatic pain, heart disease, anxiety, premature ageing – are all linked with our routine, sedentary way of life. These disorders can with justification be called the hypokinetic (or 'under-activity') diseases.

During the last few decades there has been a marked decline in our level of physical activity. Children who would once have walked three or four miles to school now travel the distance by bus. Youngsters who would have spent their weekends and summer evenings climbing trees, fishing and playing football are now immobilized in front of a TV screen. Social status demands that all adults should aspire to pursue non-manual office jobs. Technology provides us with labour-saving gadgetry as one of its major goals. We have machines to brush our teeth, grind our coffee, polish our shoes, carve our meat and open our cans of baked beans. Automation has even entered the boudoir, in the guise of phallic-shaped vibrators, designed to take the effort and uncertainty out of lovemaking. Mechanization has overtaken our games and sports, with the development of such travesties as electric golf carts and motorized pogo sticks. Thanks to the ingenuity of scientists most of our lives can now be ruled from a cushioned throne. In the morning an electric tea-maker will spare us the need to get out of bed and brew a cup of tea. In the evening, with the aid of a remote control channel selector, we can change TV stations without stirring from our chair. And if we choose, we can even exercise the dog without quitting the fireside, providing we install the latest Japanese-made automatic dog-walker with its mechanically driven conveyor belt.

Looking to the future we are offered the promise of a

yet more sedentary existence, with shopping done by remote control and journeys to work rendered obsolete by the installation in the home of computer terminals and closed-circuit television. In tomorrow's electronic world our legs could soon become an endangered species. Realizing this threat, many people are becoming physical fitness freaks and eagerly jumping on to the bandwagon of every latest health cult. One year they take out a subscription to a gymnasium, the next they join a tennis club or take up jogging. But this doesn't solve their fundamental problem. They still lead inactive lives on to which they try to graft a little irksome exercise, which is easily forgotten when work piles up, the weather's bad, they move house or they have other things to do. In this respect they are like the cranks who live on a denatured diet, stripped of most of its content of roughage and natural goodness, then rush round to the health food store to buy supplies of bran and vitamin pills. In the same way exercise buffs invest in power saws and electric pumps to inflate their car tyres, then trek round to the sports goods store to buy a static bicycle to replace the exercise which they have so carefully eliminated from their daily lives.

But this is not the only deficiency from which we suffer. In addition to being steadily deprived of physical activity, our lives have also been shorn of much mental stimulus. Compared with our primeval ancestors, our daily routines lack variety, excitement and challenge. Autocratic governments care for us from the cradle to the grave. Bureaucrats take over much of the responsibility for managing our lives. In our nine-to-five jobs week follows week with unending monotony. Housed in our neon-lit, urban pens, day blends imperceptibly into night and we become scarcely aware of the changes of the seasons or the vagaries of the climate. We no longer indulge in spontaneous play, but buy units of pre-packaged entertainment. The realities of life are not those things that happen to us from dawn to dusk, but the events we read about in the papers and watch on TV. We have become sleeping partners in the business of life rather than executive directors. As a result the besetting psychic ailments of the age are not hysteria and mania, but depression, boredom and apathy. To an ever-increasing extent our contemporary way of life is making us mentally moribund and physically effete. This is the fundamental sickness of the age.

We desperately require something to reanimate our lives. This stimulus can be provided by sudden catastrophe. Experience shows that when the interest and energies of people are mobilized during times of war, their physical and mental health invariably improves. But this is hardly a practical solution to the problems of hypokinetic disease. What we need, as psychologist William James observed many years ago, is a 'dynamogenic agent ... a moral equivalent of war'. James was no doubt thinking at the time of a revolutionary pep-pill – a multipurpose, wakey-wakey happiness drug. This the modern pharmaceutical industry is still desperately trying to find. So far, though it has tapped several rich sources of revenue, it hasn't unearthed a stimulant, tranquillizer or anti-depressant drug which is free of serious side effects. In any case while chemical potions may be able to palliate some of the symptoms of hypokinesis, they cannot possibly cure the underlying malady. If lack of exercise makes your back stiff and aching, the discomfort can be relieved by analgesic drugs, but these will not restore the lost flexibility of your spinal joints. If a deficiency of mental stimulus has made you apathetic and depressed, you may well draw a veil over your symptoms by taking anti-depressant drugs, but this will not eradicate the fundamental unhappiness of your life. The only way to overcome the hypokinetic sickness is to make a fundamental change of lifestyle. What is needed is not a dynamogenic drug, but a dynamogenic way of life.

The past few decades have seen a rapid succession of

health cults. Either they have treated the body (like weight-lifting, jogging and isometrics) or they have ministered to the mind (like transactional analysis, scientology and est). But human beings cannot be treated in this segmented way. Nor can relief be found from patchwork cures – here a crash slimming diet, there a quick course of faradic muscle toning or a few classes in bioenergetics. Health can only be procured by treating the body as an integral unit.

The body contains within itself all that is necessary for the maintenance of health. We suffer illness when the pattern of our lives is pathological; we enjoy good health when our way of life is physiologically sound. Our fundamental need today, therefore, is not for more effective therapies and drugs, but for the establishment of more efficient habits.

At present we have a simple choice. Either we continue to suffer the penalties of hypokinesis, mitigated where possible by palliative treatments and drugs, or we enjoy the positive benefits of a more dynamic approach to life. The alternatives are clearly portrayed in the diagram.

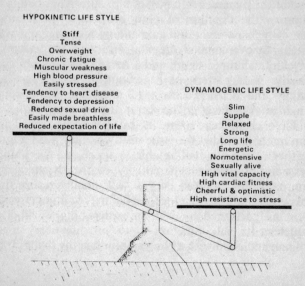

HYPOKINETIC LIFE STYLE

Stiff
Tense
Overweight
Chronic fatigue
Muscular weakness
High blood pressure
Easily stressed
Tendency to heart disease
Tendency to depression
Reduced sexual drive
Easily made breathless
Reduced expectation of life

DYNAMOGENIC LIFE STYLE

Slim
Supple
Relaxed
Strong
Long life
Energetic
Normotensive
Sexually alive
High vital capacity
High cardiac fitness
Cheerful & optimistic
High resistance to stress

For centuries disciples of hatha yoga have endeavoured to awaken the vital force in man, which they have always represented as a sleeping serpent coiled at the base of the spine, called *kundalini*. Modern medical research has failed to reveal the existence of this esoteric Loch Ness monster, but has confirmed the urgent necessity of arousing man's dormant powers. Most of us are living at a level far below our full potential. As a result of recent discoveries we now know much more about how this endless store of energy can be tapped. This vital information is described in detail in the pages of this book.

The book begins with a discussion of the nine most common expressions of hypokinetic sickness, a chapter each being devoted to fatigue, depression, anxiety, rheumatism, obesity, heart disease, lack of success, premature ageing and sexual dysfunction. But these disorders are not treated as separate entities. The treatment for one is the treatment for all – the establishment of a healthy, vital pattern of living. As psychologist Abraham Maslow once observed, 'All desirable traits in a human being correlate positively.' This is undoubtedly true of the dynamogenic way of life. Alter your habits to improve the function of your heart and you'll automatically lose weight and gain energy. Change your way of life to overcome depression and as a bonus you'll develop a slimmer figure and a more satisfying sex life. Modify your pattern of behaviour to achieve greater success and in the process you'll overcome your chronic tiredness and discover the secret of perpetual youth.

These claims may seem fanciful at this stage, but I ask you not to prejudge the issue until you have read a little further. Then you will be able to appreciate the soundness and fundamental simplicity of the dynamogenic approach. As you read on you will quickly realize that this book is not written for food faddists or fitness freaks. Nor is it designed to turn its readers into world-class athletes. Its sole function is to provide every man, woman and child with a blueprint for healthy living. It is, if you like, a commonsense manual for survival in the industrial age. It shows how you can achieve vibrant health by making slight changes in the way you eat, work, sleep and play.

After all, why be fat if it's just as easy to be slim? Why die prematurely from heart disease when a slight modification in your lifestyle could keep you climbing mountains in your eighties? Why be stiff when you can just as readily be supple? Or, as the next chapter debates, why be perpetually tired when you can equally well be overflowing with energy?

2

More Bounce to the Ounce

Are you perpetually tired? Do you sometimes wake up in the morning more exhausted than when you went to bed? Has your urge to 'get up and go' got up and gone? If so, you are not alone.

Persistent fatigue is one of the most common contemporary complaints. One physician who has made a special study of the problem finds that the lives of fully half her patients are blighted by fatigue. According to Dr Marion Hilliard, formerly chief of obstetrics and gynaecology at the Women's College Hospital, Toronto, fatigue is the greatest enemy a woman ever faces. When carried to its extreme, she says, fatigue can shorten her life or lead to mental illness. It will sap her strength and leave her at the mercy of transient infections. It can break her marriage by turning her into a shrew. Most terrible of all, it robs her of the joy and vitality without which life is grey and meaningless.

What is the cause of this chronic tiredness which drains our lives of excitement and zest? It is not poverty, for most chronically fatigued patients have sufficient money to take generous holidays and stock their homes with an endless array of labour-saving gadgets. It is rarely overwork, for most ennervated individuals will admit when quizzed that their lives are remarkably easy and routine. So why their perpetual fatigue? The answer invariably lies in their lifestyle. People are chronically tired today because their lives lack stimulus, variety and vigorous physical activity. We fall asleep in the evening because there is nothing to keep us awake, apart from the hypnotic flickering of the TV screen. Young typists claim to be so tired after a day's work that in the evening they can only summon up enough energy to collapse in a chair, eat, take a bath and tumble into bed. But what if the current boyfriend phones to invite them out to a disco party? They admit that they'd have no difficulty finding energy for such an occasion. Under those circumstances they'll happily dance the night away and still feel fresh for more. Obviously these girls are not tired, but bored. At a time in their lives when they should be bubbling over with vitality, they are allowing their inner fires to be quenched by the damp blanket of ennui.

In the sedentary age in which we live, the vast majority of chronically tired people need not extra rest, but more exercise. To remain healthy, the body needs activity just as much as it needs food and water. Without it we become feeble, tired and depressed.

It is true that fatigue can sometimes be caused by medical disorders such as anaemia, diabetes, emphysema or thyroid deficiency, but in four out of every five cases the condition is purely functional in origin. It arises largely because of the inefficient way in which we operate our body/mind machine. Learn to use your body wisely and you can maintain a persistently high level of energy output with a minimum of fatigue. Here are several ways in which this can be achieved:

- *Work at a steady pace.* Machines work most efficiently when they're operated at their optimum cruising speed. A car will give many more kilometres per litre at 80 km/h (50 mph) than when it's driven flat out at 150 km/h (93 mph). You too will function more economically if you discover your optimum pace of work and make a practice of always operating at that speed. Never let yourself be hurried. The maxim 'More haste, less speed' applies to all forms of prolonged endeavour. A distance runner may be able to run a hundred metres in well under eleven seconds, but would be extremely foolish to sprint at that pace during any part of a marathon race. If you want to be a stayer, set a pace you know you can maintain.

● *Work with minimum effort and maximum ease.* Skilled peformers can always be detected by the easy grace of their movements. There is no wasted energy or superfluous movement in the relaxed, power-packed swing of the professional golfer. No tension or jerky actions mar the fluid movements of the international tennis star. And the Grand Prix racing driver is invariably a model of relaxed composure as he comes out of a tight chicane and accelerates into the straight. How different the performance of the average weekend motorist who sits gripping the wheel, teeth clenched, brow furrowed, chin thrust aggressively forwards, as if the car were being driven by muscle power rather than horsepower. No wonder that after a brief drive in this tense state he feels as if he has just completed twenty-four hours on the Le Mans circuit. Screwing up your eyes won't help you add up a row of figures. Clenching your fists when you're late for an appointment won't make the bus you're in travel any faster, and fidgeting merely wastes energy, tests having shown that if you fidget while performing a job your consumption of oxygen can soar by as much as 80 per cent.

● *Intersperse your day with regular pauses for rest.* Laboratory tests show that the most effective way of carrying out a task is to break it up into intervals of work interspersed with regular periods of rest. This is the physiological pattern of work. It is only in this way that the human heart can keep in ceaseless action, pumping some fifty million gallons of blood during the course of an average lifetime. To avoid fatigue, the activity of the heart is organized in such a way that a short period of contraction (systole) is followed by a longer period of relaxation (diastole), during which time the cardiac muscle can rest and recharge its store of energy. A similar arrangement enables the powerful muscles of the back to keep the trunk erect during long periods of standing without tiring. This is achieved by organizing the muscle fibres into separate functional units which operate in turn rather like a gang of navvies – one group working while the others relax. In this way no section of the muscle is worked to the point of fatigue.

Generally speaking the more frequent the breaks we take, the less the fatigue and the greater the work output. This can be shown by experiments with an ergograph. In one test volunteers were asked to finger-lift a six-kilogram weight under three different operating conditions. In the first instance they were required to lift the weight at two-second intervals until they were too tired to carry on. Working in this way they generally managed to raise the weight about thirty times before they became fatigued, and then took an average of two hours to recover fully. This means that in the course of an eight-hour working day they could lift the load no more than 120 times. Their performance improved considerably when they were required to rest after every fifteen lifts. Under these conditions they got far less tired and needed only half an hour to recuperate, which meant that during an eight-hour stint of work they could lift the load 240 times. Better still was their performance when they were allowed to take a ten-second pause between each lift. Working at that steady pace they never reached the point of fatigue and could carry on working without a break, lifting the weight a maximum of 2,400 times in eight hours – a twenty-fold improvement in performance.

Dynamic individuals instinctively follow this pattern of work. Thomas Edison, the prolific American inventor who is credited with creating the phonograph, the incandescent lamp, the carbon telephone mouthpiece and over a thousand other devices, achieved his prodigious work output by taking frequent rest breaks. According to his wife, 'He was nature's man'. He worked in his laboratory until he began to feel tired, then moved into the house, snuggled down on a couch and fell asleep instantly. After three or four hours' untroubled sleep he would wake naturally, totally refreshed and eager to return to his work. Napoleon Bonaparte's enormous capacity for work can also be ascribed to his habit of taking regular periods of rest between periods of intense activity. As he himself explained, 'When I have done with one subject, I close the correspondence drawer and open another so that my various jobs never overlap one another and there is neither mental confusion nor fatigue. And when I feel sleepy I shut up all the drawers and fall asleep at once.'

● *Get adequate sleep*. Both Edison and Napoleon were wise enough to take a nap whenever they felt in need of physical rest. Many people fail to take this natural break. They ignore the promptings of the body and go on burning the midnight oil long after they should have retired to bed. If you are chronically tired and habitually get less than seven hours' sleep a night, this may be the cause of your problem. Try for a while to sleep for eight hours a night and you'll probably lose your exhaustion.

A study of a group of Canadian senior citizens showed that individuals who got less than seven hours' sleep a night were more prone to suffer from anxiety, tension and fatigue than those who normally slept longer. For a month these sleep cheats were encouraged to sleep an extra two hours a night. At the end of this period they all felt better, their complaints of tension, fatigue and anxiety had lessened and they had more vitality to cope with their daily activities.

In many cases, fatigue has a high psychological component. Tiredness is frequently used as a socially acceptable excuse for avoiding unpleasant chores. A man may profess to be too exhausted to mend a broken fuse, a wife too tired to make love, a school child too whacked out to do his homework. This defensive ploy has been used by several eminent men. 'When faced with work, Samuel Johnson was sometimes so tired, languid and inefficient that he could not distinguish the hour upon the clock,' said Boswell, his faithful chronicler. Charles Darwin also relapsed into a state of profound fatigue whenever he was faced with long journeys, painful public appearances or difficult schedules of work.

Mental fatigue also stems from apathy, boredom and lack of stimulation. If you think this may be the root cause of your problem, try taking the following steps:

● *Think positively.* If we choose to, we can think ourselves into a state of fatigue, just as we can talk ourselves into being depressed, unsuccessful or unlovable. William James, the world-famous psychologist, was one of the first people to write about this curiously negative state of mind. Most of us recognize symptoms of fatigue at some time during the day, but this is generally a subjective feeling which bears little relationship to our true physiological state. Often, according to James, we claim to have reached our self-imposed fatigue point long before we have got to the stage of true exhaustion. As he wrote, 'Some of us are really tired, but far more of us would not be tired at all unless we had got into a wretched trick of feeling tired.' Our mind responds to the signals it receives from the body. In the evenings we close our eyes, heave a weary sigh and slump heavily into a chair – behaviour which the mind interprets as evidence of bodily fatigue. If, instead of doing this, we held our bodies erect and imagined that we were like a tiger ready to leap into action, we would banish the feeling of tiredness and immediately feel fresh and alert. As James pointed out, the moods we feel are not disembodied states of mind, but the summation of stimuli coming from the body. We do not tremble because we are frightened – we feel frightened because we tremble. Our bodies are not relaxed because we are in a cheerful frame of mind. We feel cheerful because our bodies are relaxed and transmit messages to the brain which signal harmony, peace and ease. Without the relevant bodily changes – the flushed face, the tears, the muscle tension and the pounding heart – it would be impossible to experience anger, terror, love or grief. Gain mastery over the body, and you immediately establish a measure of control over the mind. Act tired and you'll feel tired. Behave as if you'd just come back from a refreshing stay at a health farm and you'll feel as lively as a wagonload of monkeys.

● *Breathe deeply.* At rest, we use only a fraction of our total lung capacity. When we're carrying out desk work, our respiration may fall to a tenth of its maximum capability. Shallow breathing of this order can lead to a state of mental torpor if it is long continued. To overcome this self-inflicted lassitude, make a habit of breathing deeply at regular intervals during the working day. Follow the yoga pattern of breathing (*pranayama*). Begin by breathing out deeply to empty the lungs of stale air. This is most important, for just as an ocean-going liner needs to empty its water storage tanks before it can take on supplies of fresh water, so we need to drain our lungs of devitalized air before we can take in an oxygen-rich replacement draught. Having exhaled fully, breathe in steadily and deeply to the count of one, hold the breath for the count of four, then exhale to the count of two. By holding the breath in this way the air is held longer in contact with the lungs' respiratory surfaces, a practice which laboratory tests show can increase the oxygenation of the blood by as much as 25 per cent. This can prove remarkably exhilarating if continued for two or three minutes, for although the brain makes up only two per cent of the body's weight, it requires 23 per cent of our total intake of oxygen. However, if you do too much deep breathing, you may find you become dizzy. Take it slowly at first. (For further details of breathing exercises see pages 266–9.)

● *Live a varied life.* Mental fatigue often occurs because one small part of the brain is overtaxed, while every other region remains fresh and under-utilized. The solution to this dilemma is to change your mental focus from time to time. After several hours spent poring over bills, bank statements and cheque counterfoils, you may be too exhausted to carry on preparing your annual tax returns, but not too tired to paint, listen to a debate on the radio, write poetry or compose a letter to a friend. In fact, indulging in these alternative activities will almost certainly provide greater refreshment than flopping wearily on to a couch.

Psychologist Henry James made a conscious point of following this practice. At one time he noted in his diary that he was simultaneously studying Sanskrit, geology, acoustics, the French Revolution, electo-dynamics and the philosophy of Charles Pierce. If his brain grew tired of pondering over the mechanism of glacial erosion and terrestrial sedimentation, he could turn the pages of his mind and switch at once to the policies of Robespierre, the Revolutionary Tribunal and the *Ancien Régime*. In this way, he overcame monotony and kept his brain alive and alert.

● *Avoid indecisiveness.* Few things are more tiring than the agony of indecision. We can exhaust the batteries of our mental computer trying to find an answer to the great imponderables of life. Should I change jobs? Should I ask for a rise in salary? Should I buy a new car? Should I tell my spouse that I'm having an affair? Far more energy is often spent in solving these dilemmas than in carrying out the deeds themselves. We may worry for months over the decision as to whether or not to send our children away to boarding school, and still not resolve the issue. Our minds become like a gramophone record stuck in its groove, going round in the same circles, repeating the same tune, but getting nowhere. On these occasions we need to give our brains a jolt to get them out of the rut. In these situations, any action is likely to be better than none. If the first step you take proves disastrous, it can generally be corrected. If you make no move at all the impasse can never be overcome. Better to waste a little energy by running initially in the wrong direction than to exhaust yourself standing still. If you're afraid to make the occasional mistake, you won't make anything. And if you genuinely don't know which way to turn, let your course of action be determined by the flip of a coin. Better that than paralysed indecision.

● *Formulate clearcut aims.* Animals that have no purpose for being up and about tend to remain relaxed and somnolent. They spring into life only when they want to fulfil a need – to assuage their hunger, to mate, play, run from their foes or satisfy their curiosity. The same principle governs human behaviour. If we're protected, well fed, comfortable and adequately entertained – as most of us are today – there's no reason for us to indulge in sudden bursts of activity. In our cossetted state we remain like well-fed cats, cosy and somnolent. For large parts of our lives we suffer in this way, from what psychologists refer to as 'motivational fatigue'. We find it exceedingly difficult to get up in the morning unless, of course, we're about to depart on a long-awaited holiday, work being less of a spur than a fortnight's trip to Paris. We're exhausted when we get home in the evening unless we're going to a party, when we're prepared to put our foot down on the throttle and tap our pent-up stores of energy. Power follows purpose. Find the reason and you'll find the means. The distinguishing feature of individuals with an enviably high output of energy is not an abnormally strong constitution, but a burning desire to achieve their aims. Many have been physically weak but have had the ability to harness every ounce of energy to help them reach their goals, like Florence Nightingale, who was a delicate child but overcame her physical handicap once she was gripped by a burning passion to improve the nursing care of the sick.

The only long-term solution to motivational fatigue is purposeful activity.

● *Keep active and purposefully occupied.* Intensive brain-work and physical inactivity are uneasy bedfellows. When we are engaged in mental work our brains require a rich supply of oxygenated blood. This supply of nourishment can be difficult to maintain in the sitting position, for at rest our circulation becomes more sluggish and our breathing increasingly shallow. Because of this, the brains of sedentary workers often tire more rapidly than they should. This can be countered by interspersing periods of brain-work with periods of vigorous physical activity. This was appreciated by the Greeks, whose peripatetic philosophers found it easier to think and debate while on the move. As Plato advised his fellow countrymen, 'Avoid excercizing either body or mind without the other.' If you're mentally fatigued, try to clear your head by running on the spot or sprinting up and down a flight of stairs. If you're too embarrassed to do this in public, retire to the nearest cloakroom and perform a series of quick calisthenic exercises. This will soon have the red corpuscles coursing to your brain, carrying with them a revivifying draught of oxygen.

Experience over the years has shown that the finest cure for nervous exhaustion and fatigue is graduated physical exercise. Visiting a beauty farm and having the body pampered with scented oils, friction rubs and whirlpool baths may be pleasurable and temporarily relaxing, but it doesn't achieve any permanent improvement in vigour. Long-term vitality is found only in action – it can't be bought in bottles. Despite this fact, vast sums of money are spent each year on tonics, pick-me-ups, brain foods and restoratives. Among the current favourites are the high-protein foods with their high-falutin' claims to be an instant source of high energy, which can do no more to banish fatigue than an omelette or a glass of malted milk. The same applies to glucose which, despite its magical reputation, provides the body with no more energy than any other sugar. Glucose may taste less sweet than cane sugar and so be more easily tolerated by invalids, and it's also slightly more rapidly absorbed within the body than the more complex molecules of fruit and cane sugars, but these qualities do nothing extra to banish fatigue or promote vitality. If your blood sugar level is low, you'll find that eating a tasty jacket-baked potato topped with a knob of butter will do as much to raise your flagging spirits as swallowing energy-packed glucose tablets. Nor will you derive much life from swallowing handfuls of multi-vitamin tablets. They're a tonic only for the directors and shareholders of the pharmaceutical companies. Providing you're on a reasonably balanced diet, which includes plenty of meat, fish, dairy foods, wholegrain cereals, fresh fruits and green, leafy vegetables, you're unlikely to be running short of any essential nutrients. (See pages 249–51 for further details of the dynamogenic diet.)

Doctors who have studied the subject report that fatigue is rarely due to dietary deficiencies, but frequently the result of insufficient physical activity. Dr Walter A. Alvarez, for many years Professor of Medicine at the University of Minnesota, noted that the fatigue of many of his patients lessened as the day wore on. 'Work, instead of making it worse, often relieves it,' he commented. This he also found true in his personal experience. 'Many a time when I myself have been so weary I wondered how I could finish my day's work, a telegram or letter full of good news or an interview with an interesting patient has swept all the fatigue away and left me feeling full of health and energy.'

Middle-aged men and women who succumb to the sedentary sickness – tiredness, fatigue and apathy – will find an injection of high-vitality living more effective than shots of Vitamin B_{12}. Instead of dosing themselves with sleeping pills and tranquillizers, they should throw open the windows of their lives to new experience. They should climb mountains, explore remote forests, ford streams and swim in turbulent seas. Sluggish bodies need stimulation, not sedation.

When weary businessmen visited Dr John Kellogg's famous sanatorium at Battle Creek, Missouri, they were quickly given something to do. Sampling the doctor's celebrated breakfast cereal was not enough. To overcome their lassitude and regain their vitality they had to take an active part in their cure. Some were set to work on simple manual tasks such as gardening. Others were encouraged to participate in crafts such as weaving, pottery and carpentry. Then there were the long country walks, the exercises in the gymnasium and the hours spent operating one of Dr Kellogg's favourite inventions – the surge bath. This was a submerged rocking chair, which had to be kept in constant motion despite the not inconsiderable resistance of the water. The general principle of the doctor's treatment was: if you want to be less tired, get tired more often. Most people can recognize the difference between healthy physical fatigue and pathological nervous fatigue. After a long walk in the country you feel pleasantly weary, your muscles are relaxed, you sleep easily and you wake totally refreshed. After the nervous fatigue of an exhausting day in the office your body is tense, you have difficulty in getting to sleep and when you drag yourself out of bed in the morning you feel as if you haven't slept a wink all night. With physical tiredness you feel at peace with the world. When your tiredness is mental in origin, you feel out of sorts and irritable. Strangely enough the two conditions rarely co-exist, for physical exertion tends to dispel nervous fatigue.

Exercise therapy has also been employed at the Mundesley Rehabilitation Unit, Norfolk. Here, patients suffering from a variety of mental and physical ailments are taken for a short course of rehabilitation treatment. On the day of their arrival, even though they may have had a tiring ambulance journey, they are given a token stint of exercise which may consist of no more than a few minutes' walk up and down the corridors in carpet slippers and dressing gown. Thereafter the basic rule of the Unit is: 'Never do less today than you did yesterday, and always do a bit more if you possibly can.' All patients receive a personally prescribed schedule of graduated exercise, which includes hilly walks, bicycle rides, golf, deck tennis, medicine-ball games and bathing in the nearby sea. Great stress is placed on activity in the open air. As the physician in charge of the Unit reasons, 'I dislike eating sweets which other people have sucked and bathing in other people's bath water and equally do I dislike breathing air which has already rinsed other people's lungs.' On this regime of vigorous outdoor exercise, known affectionately as 'Mundesley Magic', the anxious, the depressed and the weary quickly recover their old vitality. So too do most patients recovering from heart attacks and major surgical operations, despite the fact that their average age is fifty-five and their normal stay at the recovery unit less than three weeks.

If you suffer from persistent fatigue, you can do no better than adopt the dynamogenic programme outlined in full in the final chapter of this book. Then the 'Mundesley Magic' will work for you.

3

Banish the Blues

If fatigue is the commonest complaint made to physicians, depression must surely be the most frequent symptom presented to psychiatrists. Once it was referred to as the 'English Malady', an eighteenth-century British doctor estimating that lowness of spirits, together with distempers, vapours, spleen and other nervous disorders, accounted for a third of all medical consultations at that time in Britain. Now there is no doubt that melancholia is rife throughout the entire Western world. Despite our material well-being and amazing technological progress, Western civilization has been described as a 'depressive culture'. In Britain, nearly one out of every ten people becomes significantly depressed at some time during his life, and in the United States, according to an estimate made by Dr Robert Wilson, a psychiatrist specializing in teenage psychiatric problems, the lives of fully twenty per cent of American youngsters are handicapped by pervading feelings of boredom and depression. Occasional spells of mild depression may be accepted as part of the inevitable ebb and flow of life, but not so the extensive, energy-sapping periods of black despair.

One consistent symptom of these prolonged depressive states is psychomotor retardation. When we're in a melancholic mood, we don't want to walk, eat, talk, think, make love, or even raise a little finger. Charles Lamb, a frequent sufferer from depression, gave a graphic description of this agonizing state of mental and physical torpor in a letter to a friend: 'Do you know what it is to succumb under an insurmountable daymare – a terrible lethargy . . . an indisposition to do anything, or to be anything; a total deadness and distaste; . . . an indifference to locality; a numb, soporifical good-for-nothingness; an oyster-like insensibility to passing events; a mind-stupor ... ? I haven't volition enough left to dot my i's, much less to comb my eyebrows.'

At one time, the accepted cure for melancholia was to become involved in some form of physical activity. Samuel Johnson was a lifelong sufferer from depression and discovered that he could lift his despondent moods by forcing himself to overcome his lethargy and start to act. As he told his friend James Boswell, if a man is depressed, 'let him take a course in chemistry, or a course of rope dancing, or a course of anything to which he is inclined.' The fresh wind of participation will always blow away the cobwebs of despair. Nowadays this commonsense approach is rarely taken. In our loquacious, sedentary age, we prefer talking cures. The roots of depression, we are led to believe, lie buried in the arid soil of early childhood emotional traumas. But there is a biological explanation for the disease which in many ways fits in more closely with both recent scientific research into the biochemistry of the brain, and ethological studies of despondency behaviour in animals. This evidence suggests that inactivity, far from being a symptom of depression, can in many cases be its prime cause. The reason why thousands of people in the Western world slip into periods of gloom and despondency is because they get too little activity to stimulate their brains, not because early sibling rivalry has made them feel permanently insecure, or they suffered maternal deprivation in early childhood which has left them feeling chronically deprived of love. Primitive people must be far more prone to losing their mothers during their formative years, owing to the high rates of post-puerperal mortality, and yet the reported incidence of depressive illness among them is low. The recognition of this link between depression and inactivity is not new. In 1733 an English physician, Dr Cheyne, made the observation that depression was particularly common among people whose lives were characterized by 'inactivity and sedentary occupation'. Only our current obsession with psychopathology blinds us to the realization that we have become a 'depressive culture' largely because of the increasingly sedentary nature of our lives. We do not withdraw from life because we are depressed – we become depressed because we have ceased to lead sufficiently active and adventurous lives.

Depression frequently sets in after a bereavement, in the close confinement of prison camps, during the mid-life crisis, following retirement, or through sheer boredom. At first sight these situations may appear to have little in common, but closer examination reveals that they share one feature – they are all normally accompanied by a marked decline in physical activity. Take the case of bereavement. The initial reaction of a woman to the sudden death of her husband is frequently one of anxious searching. To begin with she cannot accept his departure. As one widow reported, 'Everywhere I go I am searching for him. In crowds, in church, in the supermarket. I keep on scanning the faces.' Then, with the full realization of his departure, comes a period of stunned apathy. Searching is useless. Nothing can be done to secure the loved one's return. Life, as it has been lived before, has come to an end. So the bereaved person slips into a state of resigned helplessness and melancholic inactivity. Escape from the Slough of Despond takes place only when the wheels of life begin to turn once more. A precious partner has been lost, but life goes on, and with it all the myriad activities of everyday existence. Energy must be spent on a purposeful quest to build a new life, not in a futile attempt to restore the dead to life.

Mourning is a natural response to bereavement. It becomes pathological only when the period of depressed inactivity is allowed to persist. This was better controlled in the past, when society laid down a specific time limit for the expression of mourning and grief. The Jewish tradition prescribed a seven-day *shiveh* period of strict mourning, after which the bereaved were encouraged to resume their normal activities. In the Christian church, mourners were expected to grieve for three days and then throw off their sombre mood and begin to participate again in the activities of everyday life. Now there is no generally accepted limit to the mourning period. As a result the bereaved, in an excess maybe of zeal, remorse, bitterness, guilt or rage, may withdraw from life for months on end. As a result of this self-imposed abnega- tion they enter a state of despondency and gloom, from which the only escape is purposeful activity. The woman who loses her husband inevitably suffers an abrupt reduction in her social activities. As a single woman she is likely to be invited to fewer dances and dinner parties. Without a husband she has no one to cook for, talk to, row with, or provide for. In one fatal blow she has lost not only a close companion, but also a key player in the intimate drama of her life. She suffers depression during the period of mourning because the curtain is suddenly rung down on her activities and the play is dramatically brought to a halt. She recovers her old zest the moment she realizes that the show must go on, and bravely decides to raise the curtain on the next scene.

Studies of prison inmates show a similar close link between inactivity and melancholia. Long-term convicts become apathetic if they allow themselves to be over- whelmed by the hopelessness of their plight. If they feel there is nothing they can do to improve their position, they become dejected. But experience shows that they can raise their mood by taking up a fresh hobby, following a course of study, pursuing a system of body- building exercises, waging a campaign to draw attention to their predicament, fighting to obtain an early release, or even trying to escape. The same applies to political internees and prisoners of war. Teaching recruits how to endure the rigours of solitary confinement without suffering mental breakdown or serious depressive illness is now an important part of military training. Careful interrogation of American servicemen returning from prisoner of war camps in North Vietnam showed that most had suffered at some time during their internment from periods of depression, listlessness and apathy. Investigation revealed that the most successful way of surmounting these debilitating moods was through physical exercise, establishing communication with fellow prisoners, watching insects, inventing things, playing games, maintaining health and hygiene or matching wits with the guards. The least useful survival tactics were to adopt a mien of listless resignation, contemplate suicide, or talk to oneself. Once again inactivity was found to predispose to depression, whereas purposeful mental and physical activity led to a lightening of the mood. According to the scientists conducting this study, the best way of helping prisoners with severe 'Apathy Reactions' is to coax them on to their feet and persuade them to do something, however trivial, to ameliorate their condition. The same applies to people suffering from severe depressive reactions to other stressful life situations.

Many men plunge into a decline when they reach middle age. Their friends often attribute this to the mid-life crisis, and many doctors blame it on the 'male menopause'. But as there is no evidence of an abrupt change in hormonal output at this time of a man's life, and since he has no menses to come to a pause, this seems a poor excuse for his lowered spirits. What he is often suffering from is not a shortage of hormones but a deficiency of vitality, brought about by boredom and a growing sense of the purposelessness and futility of his life. What a man or woman cries out for at this time of life is stimulus. What they are often given is sedation. Psychoanalyst Erik Erikson defines the central problem of the middle years as a conflict between generativity and stagnation. The middle-aged woman has given birth to her children, has reared them carefully and seen them safely flee the nest. What is there left for her to achieve?

At the same age her mate has probably reached the pinnacle of his career and realizes that his major goals have either been reached or proved unattainable. What remains to drive him on? If at this watershed in life a man or woman fails to find an answer to these fundamental questions they are liable to fall prey to melancholia. They are not suffering from physical debility, but from what the Germans picturesquely refer to as the *torschlusspanik* – the panic of the closing door. Trapped in this predicament they can either remain prisoners of their own hopelessness and despair, or break free from their self-imposed confinement and open the door to a new, exciting and vigorous way of life. Depression will be their constant companion if they lack the enterprise to act with novelty and verve; zest and renewed vitality will be their reward if they have the courage to accept different challenges, explore new avenues and pursue fresh goals.

Dr George Sheehan, the eminent New Jersey cardiologist, found what many might consider an unusual solution to the mid-life crisis. At a time when most men are happy to view life from a fireside chair, Dr Sheehan decided to take up marathon running. In his book *Running and Being* he tells how this happened. Like many successful men, he reached a watershed in his life – a time when 'that passion for profession or career' had changed, as Jung predicted, first to becoming a duty and now to being a burden. At this crossroad in their careers, many middle-aged men resign themselves to a life of broken dreams, failing faculties and unfulfilled ambitions. Not so Dr Sheehan. He realized he had a choice: either he could slowly relinquish his hold on life, or he could go out and grasp it with both hands. To decide his exact course of action he asked himself the simple question: 'You have only one life to live. How do you want to live it?' His remarkable reply was: 'as a distance runner.' With total dedication he vowed from that moment on to make running his vocation and medicine his avocation. 'With that decision,' he reports, 'I

33

awakened that passion, relived my dream, recaptured my youth . . . . I came to know my body and enjoy it. Things that previously exhausted me were no longer an effort. Where once I fell asleep in front of the TV set, I was up roaming the house looking for things to do. I was living on a different plane.'

Marathon running may not be your idea of a practical solution to the mid-life blues, but everyone can find relief from boredom and despondency by adopting the dynamogenic programme outlined in this book. The middle years are not a time for giving up, but a time for taking up. With the passage of every decade after the age of forty, everyone should adopt a new hobbby, pursuit or sport. This particularly applies to women who, being normally the less active sex, are most prone to depression. (In Britain the incidence of depressive illness is twice as high in women as it is in men.) The same is true of the elderly who, as they become less active, become more liable to suffer the psychological penalties of hypokinesis – boredom and depression. (This is in direct contrast to most other mental maladies, such as schizophrenia and the neuroses, which become less prevalent during the second half of life.)

Further confirmation of the hypokinetic theory of depression is provided by numerous animal studies and experiments. When deprived of their mothers or mates most animals show a grief which closely parallels the mourning behaviour of humans. Again it is noticeable that depression sets in only when grief subdues the normal desire to explore, hunt, eat, gambol and play; and recovery takes place as soon as these everyday activities are resumed. Konrad Lorenz, the father of modern ethology, has made a close study of the bereavement responses of the Greylag goose. As he reports, 'The first response to the disappearance of the partner consists of the anxious attempt to find him or her again. The goose moves about restlessly by day and night, flying great distances and visiting all places where the partner might be found.' This touching description of the frantic search to find a recently deceased loved-one bears a remarkable resemblance to the experience of the widow described earlier in this chapter. So too does the subsequent behaviour of the mourning goose. Once it realizes that searching is useless, the bereft bird withdraws from purposeful activity and becomes silent and morose. It regains its normal buoyant demeanour only after a lapse of time, when it has had a chance to adjust to the loss of its partner, and feels ready to resume its normal activities. This sequence of responses closely follows that seen in humans. Here too the initial phase of frantic searching is accompanied by a feeling of angry agitation; the period of inactive withdrawal by feelings of deep depression; and the slow resumption of customary activities with a gradual lightening of the mood. In both cases the state of mind we recognize as depression goes hand in hand with a lowered state of bodily activity. When the inertia is overcome, the despondency automatically disappears.

This relationship has also been observed in animal experiments. A state of physical listlessness, accompanied by outward signs of depression, can be induced in animals by placing them in artificially contrived situations which make them feel hopeless and helpless. Psychologists have carried out experiments with a shuttlebox – a large cage with an electrified grid floor at either end, separated by a low barrier in the centre. With the aid of this device, dogs can be trained to jump over the central partition to avoid an electric shock supplied at either end of the box. A conflict situation can be induced if both sides of the barrier are electrified at the same time. The dogs then sink into a state of apathy because they realize that no action on their part can relieve their painful predicament. From this point it is difficult to get them to take any positive action to improve their lot. Even when the opposite end of the box is not electrified and they are offered food rewards and coaxed by experimenters to cross the central divide, they still remain passive and despondent. They have entered a state psychologists refer to as 'learned helplessness'. This is the plight of many depressive patients. As a result sometimes of experience in early childhood they get the feeling that nothing they do is right. Parents often give them conflicting messages and goals which place them in an impossible 'double bind' situation. They grow up with the belief that they are worthless and unlovable, because nothing they do meets with their parents' approval. As adults they frequently show an ambivalence towards their mates. If they openly express their love and dependency towards them they feel vulnerable and easily hurt. Like moths, they know that if they allow themselves to be attracted to the candle's flickering flame they will get their wings burned. So they suppress both motion and emotion, and become increasingly inactive and sad. Why bother to toss the coin if you feel you're in a heads-you-win tails-I-lose situation?

Others fight to attain goals which as they approach them are seen to be as unreal and unsatisfying as a mirage. At this point some adopt more realistic life-enhancing targets, but others become so depressed that they give up the battle altogether. This passive resignation drives them deeper into the Slough of Despond.

Professor Mandler, head of the Psychology Department at the University of California, San Diego, has produced a parallel state in laboratory rats by giving them mazes to follow which have no meaningful goal or food reward. After trying for a while to pursue the puzzles to some purposeful conclusion, the rats finally realize that their action is completely futile. So they give up the pointless endeavour and sink into a state of unhappy lethargy. The same sequence of events can be observed in humans when they can see no point in their efforts, and no solution to their problems. As Professor Mandler says, 'Eventually, we become immobilized in a truly fundamental state of helplessness, unable to move, but continuously subjected to an extremely painful state of anxiety or distress that is unrelieved by any kind of organized behaviour.'

Experiments show that the only way of escaping this paralysing impasse is to take some form of positive action. The rediscovery of hope is the only answer to the problem of 'learned helplessness'. Life for depressed individuals will remain an endless succession of painful shocks as long as they continue to cower abjectly in one corner of their shuttleboxes. It is only when they have the courage to overcome the obstacles placed in front of them that they will discover that life on the other side of the fence is not as terrifying as they had feared. Only when they make a move can they gain the rewards dangled in front of them.

Biochemical studies provide additional support for the hypokinetic theory of depression. One of the most exciting psychiatric developments of recent years has been the discovery that certain naturally occurring chemicals – known as biogenic amines – play an important part in the regulation of mood. Representative of these substancess, and the most carefully researched, is noradrenaline – the neurohormone secreted by the body in response to excitement, arousal and stress. Chemical analyses of the brain tissues of animals have shown that drugs which increase the levels of biogenic amines in the brain tend to produce an elevation of mood. Typical of the drugs is iproniazid, and its second generation relatives phenelzine, nialamide and isocarboxazid. The antidepressant action of these chemicals was discovered by chance in 1951 when iproniazid, used to combat tuberculosis, was found to lead to a welcome elevation of mood in treated patients. The euphoria produced by the ancient drug cocaine, derived from the leaves of certain South American trees, is also known to be associated with an increase in the amount of biogenic amines circulating in the brain. Conversely, substances which decrease the levels of biogenic amines in contact with the brain cells tend to have a depressant effect. Typical of the second group of drugs is reserpine, used originally to treat patients suffering from high blood pressure, but found to lead to a disturbing degree of depression in one out of ten people treated. But it is not necessary to swallow antidepressant drugs or sniff cocaine to get a noradrenaline 'high'. Large quantities of this energizing hormone are released whenever we face up to our fears, take risks, chase after a bus, live excitingly, or introduce a measure of novelty and change into our daily routine. This no doubt explains why the incidence of depressive illness falls in times of national adversity. Every country engaged in the Second World War reported a marked drop in suicide rates while the hostilities lasted, and recent experience in Northern Ireland has shown that the incidence of depression has fallen in areas of Belfast hardest hit by the civil strife, while rising in other parts of Ireland and elsewhere throughout the United Kingdom.

Riots, wars, and aggressive interpersonal squabbles are one way of raising the levels of noradrenaline circulating in the body, and putting to rout the demons of boredom and despair, but fortunately there are other, more peaceable, ways of achieving the same end. One solution is to adopt a more dynamic way of life. In some ways our physical and emotional health is being crippled by excessive cerebration. Too often we make thinking a substitute for being. Man is characteristically the thinking hominid, or *homo sapiens*. With the aid of our massively developed cerebral hemispheres, we have the unique ability to plot and plan and scheme and dream. This is the seat of our loftiest thoughts, but also the source of our most grisly nightmares. Here is the birthplace of genius, but here also is the wellspring of insanity.

Psychosomatic illness and mood disorders occur when the forebrain paralyses or upsets the normally smooth running of the hypothalamic centres of the mid-brain. The importance of this tiny area of the brain bears no relation to its size. Although little larger than the thumb, the mid-brain, or 'old' brain, as it is sometimes called, is the centre for emotional expression, mood, sleep, appetite control, motor drive and sexual activity. When left to its own devices the mid-brain regulates these vital vegetative functions smoothly and efficiently. Problems arise only when the normal balance of hypothalamic activity is disturbed by the domination of a neurotically sick cerebrum. Frigidity and impotence can arise if the cerebral hemispheres transmit messages which have no basis in reality, but arise from groundless sexual fears and phobias. Anorexia nervosa may result if the cerebrum tells the appetite-regulating centres in the hypothalamus that starvation is the one certain way of preventing sexual maturation and so escaping all its attendant problems and responsibilities. In the same way depression will occur if the forebrain decides that the future is hopeless, and so places a check on all mid-brain activities. For the maintenance of emotional health we need an active hypothalamus, untrammelled by the domination of a neurotic or excessively repressive cerebrum.

One widely held theory of mood disorders holds that depression is due to understimulation of the hypothalamus, and mania the result of overstimulation of the hypothalamus. Certainly depressive conditions are normally accompanied by a lowering of *all* the basic hypothalamic functions (mood, sleep, sex, appetite, movement and emotional expression), while in states of mania, these activities are generally raised to fever pitch. Thus when a group of manic patients were questioned, 97 per cent said they experienced a sensation of euphoria during their upswings, 70 per cent were aware of feelings of heightened self-esteem, and 74 per cent enjoyed increased sexuality. And all were hyperactive in this particular phase of their cyclothymic cycles.

If this theory is true, or even partly true, it holds out the exciting possibility that we can escape depression by increasing the level of excitation of the mid-brain. This can be done without recourse to drugs or long courses of psychotherapy by following a dynamogenic lifestyle, rich in activity, stimulus, excitement and adventure. We need not be helpless victims of fate. It is our response to misfortune that determines our mood, not the misfortune itself. Many people get fired from their jobs, lose their lovers, fall sick, grow old, become bankrupt or get divorced, but not all allow themselves to sink into the depths of melancholia as a result. When faced with misadventures like these we either fight back or capitulate. If our response is one of resignation, we become like the dogs in the psychologists' shuttlebox experiments, paralysed by our own timidity. Viewing our plight as hopeless we cower in the self-constructed cages of our mind. And the more we withdraw from life, the less we stimulate our mid-brain, and so the more lethargic and morose we become. We feel 'fed up' because there is little to stimulate the appetite centres in the hypothalamus. We become impotent because there is nothing to arouse our sexuality. Indolence may make us feel so tired that we cannot carry out even the simplest mental test, and yet psychological studies show that depressive patients suffer no loss of cognitive, perceptual or psychomotor skills. All they lack is the necessary motivation.

Sometimes people can break free from the chains of melancholia by their own active endeavours. At other times they need the encouragement of a wise counsellor or friend. The psychologists carrying out the shuttlebox experiments found that their dogs only overcame the inertia of 'learned helplessness' when they were placed on a leash and firmly led across the central divide and shown that life on the other side of the barrier was not as terrifying as they had imagined. Sometimes this had to be done fifty times before the animals overcame their depression and fear-induced inertia.

A similar process of patient re-education is often necessary to help melancholic individuals surmount their apathy and inactivity. When depressed patients visited Dr Kellogg's sanatorium at Battle Creek, Missouri, they were given the therapeutic task of gardening. His simple advice to people suffering from melancholia, given in his book *Why the Blues?* is: 'Do some good, hard muscular work every day, enough to produce slight muscular fatigue . . . but avoid exhaustion.' Some people instinctively turn to other forms of occupational therapy when they're down in the dumps. When quizzed, a group of students listed a number of techniques they found helpful in defeating bouts of melancholia, most of which involved some kind of purposeful activity. Among the remedies they cited were taking a brisk walk, seeing a funny film, dancing, listening to music, playing sports or doing a good turn for someone else. Journalist Janet Graham, when reporting the results of this questionnaire, confessed that she too resorted to exercise whenever she needed to raise her mood. 'To beat the blues, I have learnt to take action, any kind of action, rather than wallow in my own melancholia.'

This principle has also formed the basis for many folk cures for depression. In North Africa the evil spirits of despondence are often driven away by an orgy of wild, voodoo dancing. In his book *A Cure for Serpents*, Dr Alberto de Pirajino gives an eye-witness account of the treatment of a Tripolitanian girl suffering from melancholia, supposedly caused by a 'dark and evil spirit'. For hours she gyrated in a frenzied dance, encouraged by the rhythmic chanting of her friends and the insistent beating of drums, until 'a stream of foam and sweat ran down from the corners of her mouth.' At this point, when excitement had reached fever pitch, she let out a piercing shriek and flung herself to the ground. On receiving this signal, assistants of the magician conducting the exorcism ritual stripped her of her clothes and plunged her repeatedly into water. As a result of this vigorous treatment, her mood was completely changed. Shortly afterwards she was smiling and cheerfully accepting the congratulations of her friends. The extreme stimulation had enabled her to exorcize the demon of despair.

In nineteenth-century Bavaria, Father Sebastian Kneipp, the progenitor of modern hydrotherapy, treated depression similarly with a rigorous regime of cold baths and outdoor exercise. In his handbook *My Water Cure* he recounts how he helped two students who came to him in their Easter vacation complaining of insomnia, headaches, depression and extreme fatigue. 'As it was springtime, and the ground still moist and tolerably cold, I gave them the advice to spend their holidays in walking barefoot in the woods and meadows, with rapid exercise whenever they felt cold; also from time to time to stand or walk about for two to three minutes in a stream or ditch filled with water. In like manner they were told to put their arms completely in water two or three times daily.' On this invigorating regime their spirits revived. 'With renewed zest they returned to their studies, were able to perform their tasks with ease, and joyfully looked to the autumn vacation in order to resume the work of bracing their system.'

The infliction of pain is another way of stimulating the mid-brain, which can sometimes provide an effective, if uncomfortable, way of treating depression. In medieval Europe, people afflicted with melancholia were subjected to a sound whipping to drive out the evil spirits which inhabited their souls. Even today in West Africa depressed Yoruba natives are sometimes forced to undergo the ordeal of having a series of small cuts made in their scalp and wrists.

These folk remedies for depression may seem bizarre, but it is possible that the strong stimulation of the midbrain by such primitive methods as inflicting pain, taking vigorous exercise or plunging the body into cold water may have the same beneficial effect as modern shock therapy. As psychiatrist Dr William Sargant postulates in *Battle for the Mind* when discussing the mechanism of voodoo dancing cures, 'Electric convulsion therapy for depressed patients also seems to belong to this same physiological category: because here the patient's brain is excited electrically to the point of convulsion.'

By stimulating the mid-brain, we can chase away the black clouds of despair and reveal a sunnier disposition. The medieval mystics achieved a state of transcendental ecstasy by subjecting their bodies to a regime of fasting and self-flagellation. The modern-day athlete often achieves the same state during long-distance runs. Most of our synonyms for happiness bear witness to the close connection between cheerfulness and lively activity. Spontaneous movement is an essential ingredient of such terms as gaiety, vivacity, glee, merry-making, animal spirits and jollity. The same feeling of light hearted animation is converted in similes such as 'merry as a cricket', 'happy as a sandboy' and 'gay as a lark'. Cheerfulness is the reward for active participation in life.

Get the adrenalin flowing in your bloodstream and life immediately becomes more animated and joyful. This has been proved by numerous psychological experiments. For instance, a group of students were invited to watch a slapstick film after receiving an injection of either adrenalin or a pharmacologically inert placebo. Subsequent observation showed that they reacted far more uproariously to the humour of the film when they were under the influence of adrenalin. Other experiments confirm that our emotional life is heightened whenever adrenalin raises our level of bodily arousal. The more active and adventurous we become, the greater our capacity for unsophisticated fun.

People prone to depression will gain immeasurably by adopting the dynamogenic lifestyle described in detail in the final chapter of this book. From the outset they must accept full responsibility for their mood. Either they continue to sit back and wallow in despair, or they go out, take up the threads of life again and find the contentment and joy that is waiting for them. But they must not expect to make rapid progress. The habit patterns of a lifetime are not changed overnight. To begin with they may be powerless to act when their mood is low, but on days when their spirits rise they must make the first few tentative steps to resume a more normal life. Each week they must try to break another link in the shackles of boredom, apathy and aimlessness. But they must not attempt too much too soon. Each step they take on the road to recovery must be judged so that it is rewarded by a sense of achievement, rather than punished by renewed feelings of hopelessness and failure. Here are some ways in which this can be achieved:

● *When your way ahead is clear, act – don't procrastinate.* In the early part of this century, many depressives living in the south of England made a pilgrimage to the sleepy country town of Whitwell in Hertfordshire to seek the wise counsel of a much-loved family physician called Dr L. S. Barnes. His practice embraced the usual gamut of everyday medical problems, but his speciality lay in the treatment of melancholia and nervous fatigue. Such was his skill in handling these crippling complaints that patients beat a path to his door from all over Europe. With infinite patience he coaxed people to overcome their despondence and regain their health. Patients who complained that they were too tired to stand were engaged in long conversations in his garden, just to prove that their feelings of fatigue were purely subjective in origin. Their greatest foes were their own forebodings. Like mesmerized chickens they were paralysed by their own imaginings and crippled by the evil spells cast by their own subconscious minds. To these people he gave the courage to act. He told them, 'When your enemy puts up a sign: "Danger. To pass beyond this point means catastrophe", I say to you: "Go and see." Beyond that sign lie, not what you expect, but green fields and happiness. Your subconscious mind is stealing from you day by day the happiness which should be yours.' In this way he led them out of the shuttle-boxes of their minds, and gradually restored their will to live.

In the days of the great Egyptian kings indolent people were sentenced to death. Today the penalty for idleness is boredom and depression. Antidepressant drugs may provide symptomatic relief, but they can give rise to unfortunate side effects, and such is their unpopularity that they are not taken by 40 per cent of the patients for whom they are prescribed. The efficacy of psychotherapy is also open to doubt, for a study of the research literature fails to show that psychoanalysis has any beneficial effect on the course of depressive illness. Interpretative analysis alone is not enough, unless it modifies the way we act. The discovery that our deep-seated feelings of inadequacy stem from the denigrating treatment we receive in childhood does not of itself remove our sense of worthlessness. Recovery comes only when we act in ways which directly enhance our self-esteem. We rehabilitate the mind, by re-awakening the body. As psychiatrist Jack Dominian says in his book *Depression*, 'Those who like to conquer their depressive mood alone may overcome it with activity. They will forget their misery by doing something. They plunge more deeply into their work. They undertake new commitments. They carry out the age-old maxim of turning away from themselves and considering others. In the home there is always something which needs doing, such as decorating, repairing or constructing something new. The pleasure of achievement overcomes the distress of misery.'

● *Take a daily constitutional walk or run*. Many people find that they can shake off the blues by taking a

45

brisk walk. This was the remedy practised by Bertrand Russell. It was his firm conviction that 'unhappy businessmen would increase their happiness more by walking six miles a day than by any conceivable change of philosophy.' Depressive subjects can derive even greater benefit once their general health has improved by going for a gentle daily jog. Many psychiatrists have found that running is a more effective remedy for states of mild despondency than antidepressant pills. Psychiatrist Robert S. Brown, of the University of Virginia at Charlottesville, started prescribing running when he discovered that 'nobody jogging down at the track ever appeared depressed.' He estimates that depression is the presenting symptom of approximately 70 per cent of his patients, and claims that all but 15–20 per cent have shown 'quick benefit' within the first week of taking up a programme of regular running.

● *Live a varied life.* Ennui is one of the commonest causes of apathy and despondency. Our lives are becoming increasingly predictable and routine. Day follows day with little change. What occupies our time today is likely to engage our attention next week, next month and next year. Without the stimulus of change we are apt to sink into a state of mental and physical torpor. But again the choice is ours. Either we plump for the comfort and safety of the tried and tested routine, or we accept the excitement and stimulus of innovation. As psychologist Fritz Perl has pointed out, boredom involves a deliberate act of focusing attention on routines that are monotonous and mundane, while resolutely withholding attention from activities that are novel and exciting. To escape from the morass of tedium, take out a pencil and paper and make a list of the tasks you've always wanted to tackle, the places you've meant to visit, the subjects you've planned to study, the heights you've intended to scale; then set out painstakingly and methodically to achieve these goals. Don't be content to live in a world of fantasy. Set out to make your dreams come true. In this way despondency will be put to rout for, as consulting psychologist William Brown observed more than thirty years ago, 'It is extraordinary how anxiety and depression will clear up once the patient's interests are aroused in new ventures and his decision is made, without reservation to go forward.'

● *Don't be deterred by initial failure or disappointment.* Disappointment leads to depression only when we throw in the towel and quit fighting. So long as we maintain the struggle to overcome frustations and setbacks, we avoid sinking into a mood of gloomy impotence. Keep the flame of hope burning brightly and the dark shadows of despair will disappear. Teenagers often become moody and depressed when young love turns sour and their initial overtures of affection are spurned. They fail to realize that sometimes this rejection is merely a testing of the strength and sincerity of their ardour. Faint hearts like this rarely win fair ladies, and quickly become dejected.

So it is with life's other endeavours. Many people blame their despondency on an unfortunate start in life. They are content to number themselves among life's failures because they were orphaned at an early age, suffered numerous childhood illnesses or had an inadequate education. Yet this is the background of many of the world's most successful men and women. Beethoven was the offspring of a consumptive mother and an alcoholic father, Schubert the progeny of a peasant father and a mother in domestic service, and Shakespeare the son of an impoverished butcher and an illiterate woman incapable even of signing her own name. Many great statesmen were orphaned early in life. A study of the life history of British Prime Ministers from Walpole to Neville Chamberlain shows that 67 per cent of them suffered the loss of one or more parents in childhood or early adolescence. Poverty has been the breeding ground of many dictators: Mussolini was the son of an indigent blacksmith and Hitler the offspring of a poorly-paid, illegitimate customs officer who died when he was fourteen years old. Again, Charles Darwin and Winston Churchill had indifferent records at school and Albert Einstein, who didn't speak until he was four, showed so little aptitude for his studies that one of his teachers remarked, 'You will never amount to anything.' It is obviously not the start we make in life that matters, but the way we run the race. We fail and become despondent only if we remain forever rooted to our starting blocks.

An analysis of the histories of the tsars of industry shows that above all else they have had the ability to fight back from failure. The young H. J. Heinz went bankrupt early in his career, when he spent his last dime buying a horse to pull his trader's cart and the horse later proved to be blind and utterly useless for the task. Instead of accepting defeat at this point he fought back and went on to produce one of the world's largest food-producing firms. When F. W. Woolworth established his first Five-Cent Store in Utica, New York, it was a dismal flop, but he was so convinced of the soundness of the idea that he ignored this early reverse and opened another store in Lancaster, Pennsylvania, which proved an unqualified success. Out of initial defeat came the foundation of the world's largest group of chain stores. These men acquired and maintained an attitude of aggressive optimism, whereas the animals in the psychologists' laboratories became despondent and ineffectual through adopting an attitude of 'learned hopelessness'.

The success and happiness of our lives depends to a very large extent on the way we respond to temporary setbacks. This is never more true than in the field of writing. An aspiring novelist needs dogged persistence as much as a facility with words. John Creasey, the world-famous novelist who went on to sell sixty million books, had to endure the humiliation of 743 rejection slips before he had a single word printed. Richard Adams' phenomenal best-seller *Watership Down* was turned down by three literary agents and four publishers before a little-known publishing house decided to give it a small print run. And Agatha Christie's first detective novel, *The Mysterious Affair at Styles*, was turned down by publisher after publisher for three years before it finally appeared in print. Even then it sold fewer than 2,500 copies, and gained little critical acclaim for its author, who won recognition only after the publication of her seventh book.

People are not failures because they have one, two or even thirty setbacks. They become failures only when they stop trying. That's when despondency sets in.

● *Get yourself fit, and refuse to allow yourself to become a martyr to sickness.* Reactive depression often settles in after a severe and debilitating illness, but only if we let it. The curse of ill-health can be a bridle to aspiration or a spur to greater endeavour. John Milton became blind, and yet carried on to write such spellbinding poetry as *Paradise Lost* and *Paradise Regained*. Much of Beethoven's greatest music was written after he became totally deaf. El Greco and Manet suffered from severe astigmatism, but overcame their disability to become two of the world's most famous painters. Julius Caesar laid the foundation of the Roman Empire despite begin afflicted with epilepsy. Franklin Roosevelt, although crippled by polio, went on to become President of the United States. Demosthenes and Winston Churchill were handicapped by a pronounced stammer in their youth, but both triumphed over their disability to become eminent public orators.

These men refused to become resigned to a life of invalidism and despair. Some people become despondent the moment they suffer a twinge of rheumatism, others retain their optimism despite being deprived of limbs, sight, movement or hearing. Some refuse to acknowedge their handicaps. Others identify themselves with their sickness, proudly telling the world about *my* headache, *my* arthritic knee or *my* ulcer. But even severe illness needn't give rise to feelings of either hopelessness or helplessness. Blind skiers have taken part in downhill slalom races; a man with two artificial legs has climbed the formidable 13,026-foot Eiger mountain, and a paraplegic polio patient has swum twenty-five miles in his attempt to cross the English Channel. For a while, portrait painter Simon Elwes gave way to apathy and despair when a stroke paralysed his right arm and hand. He recovered and overcame his depression when he taught himself to paint with his left hand. Now he has the distinction of being the only Royal Academician who has had paintings selected for showing in the Academy's prestigious Summer Exhibition of which some are painted with the left hand and others with the right.

Deafness, debility and disease get us down only when we let them weaken our hold on life. Eddie Rickenbacker, America's most decorated pilot in the First World War, had many brushes with sickness and death. Every time he maintained his hope; always he fought back. On one occasion, at the age of fifty-one, he was seriously injured in a plane crash. Lying in hospital under an oxygen tent he heard a radio newsreader named Winchell reporting his imminent demise. The shock of this announcement gave him the will to live. 'I began to fight,' he recalled. 'They had me under an oxygen tent. I tore it apart and picked up a pitcher. I heaved it at the radio and scored a direct hit. The radio fell apart and Winchell's voice stopped. Then I got well.' Sixteen months after recovering from this injury he crashed again. Landing in the sea, he kept himself alive for twenty-one days on an open raft by killing and eating a seagull that fortuitously landed on his head. Nothing would make him give in. As he boasted afterwards, 'I've cheated the Grim Reaper more times than anyone I know, and I'll fight like a wildcat until they nail down the lid of my pine box.'

There are occasions in life when it often seems easier to die than to live. Struggling at these times may appear futile. All too easily then we allow ourselves to be slowly lowered into the inky well of despair. But even in the throes of severe debilitating illness we have a measure of control over our mood. As a polio victim replied when told by a friend that affliction colours an individual's life, 'Yes, and I propose to choose the colour.' Either we opt to wear the red badge of courage or the black drapes of resigned despondency. This even applies to our reaction to terminal illness. Dr Cecily Saunders, of London's St Christopher's Hospice, has made a special study of the management of dying patients, half of whom suffer depression during their last few weeks of life. She finds that much can be done to help these people face their death with equanimity. Analgesic drugs may ease their pain, but cannot of themselves lighten their despondency. To avoid depression, she reports, the dying patient must be 'helped not only to die peacefully but also to *live* until he dies.'

● *Be enthusiastic about all you do*. Work is for many

51

people the finest therapy for depression. A number of famous historical figures, such as Napoleon, Nelson and Goethe, suffered from periods of deep despair, but found they could conquer their mood by immersing themselves in purposeful work. As a young man, Abraham Lincoln was once so depressed that he asked his close friends to keep knives and razors out of his reach. Then he discovered a purpose for living, and embarked upon a political career dedicated to the concept of freedom and democracy which gave him no chance to be bored or more than temporarily despondent.

Even zoo animals, when gripped by monotony, will find some excuse to busy themselves. A caged mongoose, stripped of the opportunity to hunt for game, will keep itself alive and alert by 'shaking to death' a slab of dead meat. A cossetted pet cat, to pep itself up, will toss a dead mouse into the air, simply to have the fun of pouncing on it when it falls. In this way captive animals inject a little excitement into their dull, lethargic lives.

We need work to give point and purpose to our lives. Melancholic individuals are often obsessed with the aimlessness and futility of their existence. These nihilistic feelings can best be dispelled by engaging in some form of purposeful activity. Herein lies our identity, our challenge, our stimulus and our major source of satisfaction. Few people remain mentally healthy without a firm commitment to a worthwhile hobby or job. As psychologist Abraham Maslow said after a lifetime spent comparing the lives of neurotic and well-adjusted people: 'I never met a happy individual who was not committed to a job or cause outside himself.' It is the duty of the leaders of industrial societies to provide each individual with the opportunity of satisfying this basic need.

● *Let yourself go; give vent to your feelings whenever possible.* Psychiatric studies reveal that depression is often associated with repressed emotion. People become despondent because instead of acting out their feelings they turn them inwards. Psychiatrist Willem Van Dijk was asked by the Dutch government to assist in the treatment of hostages held for some days in a hijacked plane by South Moluccan terrorists. Previous experience had shown him that people subjected to severe emotional traumas such as this suffer either from highly emotional outbursts or from deep depression. The main aim of his therapy, therefore, was to provide an opportunity for emotional catharsis. Victims were encouraged to cry, talk at length about their experience, and give outlet to their pent-up emotions of aggression and fear. A similar policy was adopted recently by the twenty-five psychologists who volunteered to assist the city workers called to cope with debris of San Diego's worst-ever air disaster: They prescribed jogging, target shooting and a variety of other sports to help the workers unleash their suppressed horror and rage. As Alan Davidson, president of the Academy of San Diego Psychologists said, 'We wanted the anger to come out in an appropriate, directed way.' The word apathy stems from the greek root *a-pathos* – an absence of feeling. This gloom-ridden state arises whenever people are unable, or unwilling, to express their anger, or work through their frustrations. Again passivity is the sickness, and activity the cure.

● *Enjoy life's pleasures to the full.* Keep a list of the things that consistently give you real enjoyment and make a point of doing them whenever you're feeling low. This will encourage you to overcome your inertia, and also give you an immediate source of positive satisfaction. Bake a cake, dig the garden, visit a friend, sing a song, or go out and buy a new pair of shoes. Do anything that will raise your mood and engender a spirit of gaiety.

But whatever policy you adopt to defeat depression, whether it's occupation therapy, creative work, jogging, or emotional abreaction, it's likely to be an active rather than a passive cure. In essence the remedy will be found to lie in the precept of Alfred Lord Tennyson: 'I must lose myself in action lest I wither in despair.'

4

Begone, Dull Care!

Anxiety is one of the predominant symptoms of the modern world. Scan the faces of the crowds commuting into any city in the Western world and you'll find them etched with worried frowns and perplexed expressions. Sit in a doctor's consulting rooms and you'll hear an endless dirge of anxiety symptoms – patients whose nagging problems intrude on their sleep; young couples unable to enjoy a normal sex life because of their chronic tensions; pretty young girls with skins blemished by the unsightly stigma of nervous dermatitis; housewives whose lives are plagued with tension headaches; executives eaten up with worries to the extent that they've developed peptic ulcers. Anxiety has become one of modern medicine's greatest concerns.

To assess the prevalence of anxiety states, Dr Malvin Salkind, director of the department of general practice at St Bartholomew's Hospital, London, devised a psychological questionnaire based on interviews with a group of several thousand patients receiving treatment for nervous complaints. The quiz was designed to reveal a person's 'anxiety level', and included questions about his ability to relax, the ease with which he went to sleep at night, and whether or not he suffered from irrational fears or phobias. On collating the results, Dr Salkind found that a score of 14 represented the borderline between relative normality and states of anxiety requiring medical treatment. Interviewers then gave the questionnaire to a wide selection of people scattered throughout the British Isles. It revealed that the anxiety level of this random sample of the British population measured an average of 13.9 on Dr Salkind's scale. This suggests that vast numbers of seemingly healthy Britons are borderline sufferers from anxiety neurosis. The British public, and no doubt the population of every other industrialized nation, is obviously living on its nerves.

What is the explanation for this creeping malaise? Why are so many people today perpetually tired, tense and troubled? One reason, no doubt, is that we are being constantly bombarded by alarming news. Every time we open a daily newspaper we read accounts of hijackings, murders, rapes, muggings and audacious burglaries. When we switch on the TV, we see alarming newsreel shots of gory massacres in Africa, violent street riots in Central Europe, or the heaped corpses of famine victims. Even in our day-to-day encounters we face the same litany of woe. When we chat to chance acquaintances in the street their conversation invariably ranges from the relatively trivial woes of inflation through to the dire consequences of nationwide strikes, burgeoning street violence and the breakdown of law and order. No wonder we become anxious and tense when we're subjected to this constant bombardment of stressful sights and sounds. Like a flock of birds or a herd of cattle, we respond immediately to the distress cries of our fellows. But unlike these animals our response is purely passive. We hear the alarm call but do not react to it by taking any form of physical action. We don't take flight from the happenings that alarm us, or fight the entity that makes us afraid. We know that there is nothing we can do to help the victims of a brutal massacre in Central Africa and little we can offer to alleviate the lot of the starving masses in Calcutta. We are constantly faced with global problems like these, but can only offer a parochial cure. So we remain activated but inert, stimulated but unreleased. This is the prime cause of the chronic anxiety we suffer. We are like racing greyhounds, stimulated by the roar of the crowd, the expectancy of the race and the tantalizing movement of the mechanical hare in front of us, but held pinioned by circumstance in our traps.

Atavistic physiological changes occur within our systems whenever we're under stress. These prepare our body for protective action. When primeval man came face to face with a sabre-toothed tiger his muscles tensed, his pulse raced, his blood pressure soared, stress hormones, fats and sugar flooded his bloodstream and the clotting power of his blood was increased to staunch the bleeding that might arise in any ensuing battle. In this way he was equipped for either flight or fight. Whatever his choice of action, the stressful situation was quickly over. Either he climbed to safety up the nearest tree, clubbed the beast to death, or died in the attempt. Today's stress is different in that it often persists unchanged for long periods of time. A man at work may be at loggerheads with his boss for several years. After their first clash he feels the muscles of his neck and shoulders tense up ready to do battle. But he resists the desire to punch the man on the nose, partly out of deference to his seniority and partly because he needs to keep his well-paid job. So he continues to suffer unrelieved tension, and experiences increasing fibrositic pain in his neck and shoulders. Since he is prevented from acting out his conflict, his boss remains a permanent and literal pain in the neck.

At home a wife suffers countless slights and indignities from an uncaring husband which make her blood boil. But having been schooled to believe that nicely brought up ladies never row or make a scene, she bottles up her rage. To the outsider she may appear calm, but medical checks reveal that, with no safety valve to relieve the mounting tension in her cardiovascular pressure cooker, she is suffering from persistently high blood pressure. The motorists who dice with death each day in our concrete jungle paths suffer the same haematological changes as did Neolithic man when he was brought face to face with the terrors of the primordial forests. Tests on drivers reveal an increase in the level of fats circulating in their bloodstreams even when they are driving in a relaxed fashion over familiar territory. When the driving becomes increasingly hazardous these changes are more pronounced. Tests on Grand Prix racing drivers competing at Brands Hatch, Nurburgring and Spa reveal that the stress of competitive driving releases so much fat into their bloodstreams that while samples of their blood plasma are clear before a race, they become decidedly milky once the race is over. This primitive response is brought about by the sudden outpouring of stress hormones which mobilize the body's fat reserves and release into the bloodstream countless tiny globules of fat which provide additional fuel for muscular activity. The injection of this calorie-rich fuel is beneficial if the anxiety-provoking situation promotes immediate action, but can be positively lethal if activity is either irrelevant, inhibited or postponed. The additional calories may have powered the caveman and helped him stave off the attack of a predatory animal but they can't possibly assist the racing driver or increase the performance of his car. So the fats continue to circulate unused in his bloodstream, until they are absorbed into the blood walls where they form the telltale fatty plaques of atheroma, the basis of cardiovascular disease. This explains why the intensive care units of metropolitan hospitals throughout the Western world invariably contain more than their fair share of taxi drivers, who have to face the stress of chaotic city traffic, with little opportunity to take sufficient exercise to burn up the unwanted fats which pour constantly into their bloodstreams. Anxiety itself is not a killer, as I explained in my book *The Stress Factor*. Providing it leads to positive action, stress can enhance performance, stimulate creativity, relieve boredom, and even prolong life. It becomes dangerous only when it is unduly prolonged, or is not accompanied by some form of physical activity.

Animals appear to have an innate understanding of this biological fact. They normally respond immediately and vigorously to the promptings of their internal emotional state. They are rarely the victims of passive stress. If they're afraid, they run. If they're annoyed, they bellow with angry rage. If they feel skittish, they play. If they're trapped or frustrated, they struggle to free themselves from their limitations. If they're attacked, they fight. And if their adversary is too powerful to tackle head on, they quietly slope off from the battlefield and give vent to their fury on something else. This enables them to dissipate their anxiety without coming to any immediate or long-term physical harm. Ethologists refer to this behaviour as displacement activity. If two fighting cockerels come into direct confrontation and decide not to battle it out, they will turn away and release their energy by pecking furiously at the ground. Instead of fighting, antelopes will vent their anger on neighbouring trees; herring gulls will tug at tufts of grass and belligerent stickleback fish will stand on their heads and dig holes in the sand with their snouts. By engaging in these harmless rituals, they quickly and safely dispel their tension states.

Similar behaviour patterns are occasionally seen in humans. Anxious expectant fathers are traditionally expected to pace up and down the corridor outside the maternity ward; frustrated toddlers will throw cushions or pummel their teddybears; nervous candidates for a job will drum their fingers on a table-top while waiting for their crucial interview; and anxious examination students will doodle furiously on a scrap of paper, or fiddle with a paperclip, as they rack their brains to recall a vital fact. These are all examples of displacement activity – a socially advantageous technique for dealing with conflict situations which we could use more frequently than we do. Why rush into a precipitate row with your lover or mate if you can let off steam by felling a tree or running round the block? As Dr George Stevenson advised in a booklet issued by the US National Association for Mental Health, 'If you feel like lashing out at someone, try holding out until tomorrow. Meanwhile, pitch into some physical activity like gardening or carpentry, or golf, or a long walk. Working the anger out of your system will leave you much better prepared to handle your problem intelligently.'

Many people do this instinctively. Gertrude Lawrence, the musical comedy star who captivated audiences in both Britain and America, invariably immersed herself in a frenzy of useful activity whenever she was under stress. This enabled her to dissipate her tension without becoming either tetchy or withdrawn. Her understanding husband, Richard Aldrich, grew accustomed to her sudden sallies into organizing bazaars, lawn parties, clam bakes, community rallies and fund-raising auctions. He realized that at times she needed these outlets to ease the pressure of theatrical life. What he found difficult to accept was her predilection for risk ventures, such as flying in helicopters or embarking on deep-sea fishing excursions. But, as he perceptively deduced in his tender biography *Gertrude Lawrence as 'Mrs A.'*, 'It seems probable that by these flirtations with danger she worked off some of the emotional tension which other more temperamental stars, male and female, release through bursts of bad temper backstage and in public. Or which they appease by chain-smoking or excessive drinking.'

This is a characteristic of high vitality people – they maintain their relaxed good humour, and infectious zest for life, by keeping constantly active. Never for a moment do they allow themselves to wallow in anxious reveries or idle self-pity. They exude a bustling energy which puts to rout the butterflies of fear. Madame de Pompadour was such a person. Many people misguidedly view her simply as the beautiful courtesan of Louis XV, but in fact sex played a relatively small part in her relationship with the king. For many years the secret staircase between her boudoir and Louis' chambers was blocked up, and she encouraged him to satisfy his sexual needs with prostitutes discreetly housed in a small villa on the outskirts of Versailles. What she offered the king was a vivacious personality and the opportunity to escape while in her company from the affairs of state and all the perplexing problems of a nation in a state of rapid social change. Queen Marie was dull. An evening in her company invariably ended with a desultory game of cards and a doze in front of an open roaring fire. Even her father, the penniless King Stanislas of Poland, was forced to admit that his daughter and her mother were undoubtedly the dullest queens in Europe. 'When I'm with her I yawn like at Mass,' he openly confessed. But Madame de Pompadour was a totally different proposition. She loved to entertain, danced with passion and grace, laughed constantly and enchantingly, was a skilled clavichord player, a keen horticulturist, an avid collector of rare and exotic birds, a talented painter, and an enthusiastic producer of amateur plays in which she both acted and sang to entertain the king. As her biographer, Nancy Mitford, justifiably claims, 'Madame de Pompadour excelled at an art which the majority of human beings thoroughly despise because it is unprofitable and ephemeral: the art of living.' It was this priceless attribute that the king admired and wished to share, for he found that by partaking freely of her interests, he could leave behind his regal worries and cares. Her gay, vital way of life was the ideal antidote to the grave responsibilities of kingship. She was the perfect occupational therapist and even encouraged the king to establish in the grounds of the Palace of Trianon a miniature farm complete with farm buildings, cows and hens, so that they could escape together from time to time to lead a carefree, bucolic existence, free from the petty squabbles and irritating restrictions of courtly life and protocol.

As was explained in the last chapter, too many people today live in their heads rather than in their bodies. They experience emotions in their brain, but deny them proper physical expression. In their reveries they build castles in the air, but in reality they never even lay the foundations for their plans and schemes. In their sexual fantasies they may be wild, spontaneous, original and free, but in their actual relationship with their lovers and mates they are tense, inhibited and staid. Rather than be exposed to the uncertainties and risks of real living, they have retreated into their cerebral shells. They have made thinking a substitute for being, and have in the past been encouraged in this sterile pursuit by the general consensus of psychiatric thought. But opinion is now changing. Psychiatrists of all persuasions are gradually realizing the relative ineffectiveness of purely talking cures. Some years ago Professor Hans Eysenck, of the Institute of Psychiatry, London, followed the histories of a group of over seven thouand psychiatric patients who had received various forms of psychotherapy. He found that irrespective of the treatment they received, whether strict Freudian analysis, the Jungian technique of Analytical Psychology or any of the shorter forms of psychotherapy, approximately two-thirds of the patients recovered. This appeared to justify the use of psychotherapy, until it was discovered that the spontaneous recovery rate from neurotic illness was almost exactly the same. In fact, a review of a group of severely neurotic patients who were admitted to hospital for purely custodial care, combined with a study of five hundred people who received no psychotherapeutic treatment whatsoever but claimed disability payments from the Equitable Life Assurance Society on psychiatric grounds, showed that 72 per cent of neurotic patients can expect to enjoy complete recovery from their illness or substantial improvement within a period of two years *without receiving treatment of any kind*. As Professor Eysenck concluded, this revelation should provide a grain of comfort for the thousands of people suffering from neurotic illness, but can offer little encouragement to the psychiatrists who practise any of the many forms of purely analytical therapy. What anxious, over-stressed patients require is not an endless post-mortem of their problems, but a positive course of action to help them overcome their unhappy state of mind.

62

Millions of people throughout the world are beset by specific fears and phobias. When a team of market researchers questioned a group of three thousand Americans they found that nearly 41 per cent feared speaking in public, 32 per cent were afraid of heights and 22 per cent were petrified of insects and bugs. Many others had a dread of open spaces (agoraphobia), closed spaces (claustrophobia), blood (haematophobia), cats (ailourophobia), dogs (cynophobia), germs (bacteriophobia), pain (algophobia) or the dark (nyctophobia). Countless hours could be spent trying to discover the origin of these pathological fears, for nobody is *born* with a dread of germs or cats. In fact, when Dr John B. Watson carried out his classical experiments at the John Hopkins Maternity Hospital, Maryland, he found that newborn babies showed only two innate anxieties – a fear of loud noises, and a fear of being dropped. He discovered that infants had no inborn fear of spiders or the dark. When he took a tiny child called Albert to the zoo and confronted him at close quarters with snakes, large birds and cats he showed not the slightest quiver of concern. In fact the only response the baby showed was when a camel coughed in his face – an experience which is both unexpected, noisy and overpoweringly smelly.

This research shows that the vast majority of adult fears are acquired rather than inherited. Like Pavlov's dogs we develop a conditioned fear response, and learn to tremble when we hear the ringing of a bell, get trapped in a lift or catch sight of an inoffensive spider or mouse. Given time, we could no doubt trace the origin of these phobias to some childhood trauma. But why waste time on this largely academic exercise? Fears are learned, and must be unlearned by a process of active deconditioning.

Supposing you are petrified of spiders and at present shudder the moment one sidles in sight. Set yourself the task of tackling this unreasonable fear by easy stages. To begin with, simply imagine that a large, woolly-legged spider is crawling towards you on the floor. When you can entertain this thought with relative equanimity, equip yourself with a series of photographs of spiders, and spend time studying their anatomy, peering into their beady eyes, and examining their long, spindly legs. When this exercise no longer holds any qualms for you, get hold of a toy spider from a shop that specializes in novelty items such as fake ink stains, sneezing powder and stink bombs, and place it in your wardrobe, on the breakfast table or wherever else it's likely to have the greatest shock effect. When this ceases to make your spine creep, progress to viewing dead spiders and then to contemplating the genuine live articles with all their cold, creepy, crawling menace. In this way, by actively facing up to your anxieties, you'll put your fears to rout. As the American poet and essayist Ralph Waldo Emerson rightly said, 'Do the thing you fear and the death of fear is certain.' This applies to all the myriad other day-to-day anxieties.

Fears are like ghosts. Run away from them and they'll continue chasing you; turn and face them and they'll immediately disappear. How many of the four-out-of-ten Americans who fear public speaking have actually gone out of their way to overcome their dread? Few will have attended courses in public speaking, studied self-improvement books or seized opportunities to stand up and say a few words in public. Instead they will have harboured the fear of public speaking in the recesses of their minds, where it will have burgeoned until it has reached gargantuan proportions. The only way to overcome the fear of addressing an audience is to stand up and speak in public, and to carry on doing so until repeated practice strips the experience of its terrors. This is the technique that many of the world's orators have had to use to overcome their initial stagefright. Two of the most eloquent men in British parliamentary history, Benjamin Disraeli and David Lloyd George, suffered platform nerves at the start of their political careers. Disraeli admitted that he would rather have led a cavalry charge than deliver his maiden speech in the House of Commons, and Lloyd George confessed that when he first stood up to speak in public, 'my tongue clove to the roof of my mouth; and, at first, I could hardly get a word out.' Both these men overcame their nervous disability, not by endless introspection and self-analysis, but by pursuing a courageous course of positive, fear-abating action.

More of life's failures are caused by lack of courage than by lack of ability. We are lonely and fail to make friends not because we are intrinsically dull or unlovable, but because we shrink back from making contact with strangers. We would rather stay in our lonely shells than risk suffering a rebuff. We would dearly love to take up amateur dramatics, but don't want to make fools of ourselves in public. So we remain forever on the other side of the footlights, always watching the drama of life from the safety of the stalls. We feel we are worthy of greater responsibility at work, but lack the nerve to ask for promotion. All too often we fail to get what we want in our business or social life, simply because we haven't the guts to ask for it. As Shakespeare wrote, 'Our doubts are traitors, and make us lose the good we oft might win, by fearing to attempt.' Life is never without risks, and the person who is not prepared to make a mistake will make nothing.

The way to overcome fears and achieve success is to follow a bold course of action, fixing a definite goal and then marching resolutely towards it. This also helps to dispel the physical tensions that are the cause, as well as the result, of chronic anxiety. Most people accept the psychosomatic mechanism of disease. They acknowledge that people can worry themselves into an ulcer, headache or heart attack, but they often fail to appreciate that the reverse process also operates. There is in fact a somaticopsychic mechanism whereby pathological states of the body have an adverse effect on the mind. This is clearly seen in the relationship between mental anxiety and physical tension. When we hold our muscles tense a constant stream of information is relayed to the brain, warning it that the body is wound up and ready for emergency action. The alarm is sounded by the body's muscular outposts, and is relayed to the brain where it maintains the psychic control centre at a state of constant alert. This is a condition known to psychiatrists as 'free-floating' anxiety. In this tense, agitated mood we are perpetually on the lookout for trouble. The muscles give the message that disaster is just around the corner, and the mind keeps fretting until it finds reason to justify the body's flustered state. This is never difficult to do. When we're conditioned in this way we conjure up dilemmas which have little substance in reality. They are by any reckoning irrational fears – ghosts which can't be reasoned away or explained in strictly psycho-analytical terms. For this reason the simplest solution to the problem of free-floating anxiety is not to embark on long courses of psychotherapy or nerve-numbing drugs, but to release the tension in the body's muscles. The moment this is done the all-clear is sounded and the state of anxiety lifts. From the powerful muscles of the back through to the tiniest muscles of the hand a stream of messages flows back to the brain repeating, 'All is well. We're not ready to fight or run away from danger. The emergency is over.' So both body and mind relax. This state of repose can be induced in a number of purely physical ways. A hot bath helps, so does an overall body massage, but one of the most effective ways of achieving relaxation is to perform the Reveille Ritual described on pages 273–6. This series of movements will stretch out and ease the tension in all the body's major muscle groups. Just as the simplest way to overcome cramp in the leg is to stretch out the painfully contracted muscles, so the easiest way to achieve general relaxation is to stretch out the tense muscles of the neck, trunk and limbs. The same effect can be achieved by taking part in any form of vigorous exercise. Displacement activities of this kind will help to dissipate the tensions which haven't found outlet in other ways.

Tension-releasing exercises can also be useful in the alleviation of anxieties which have a more obvious cause. Psychiatrist Richard Driscoll, of the psychiatric hospital in Tennessee, proved this when he evaluated several different ways of treating students' pre-examination nerves. He discovered that one of the most effective ways of reducing anxiety in this situation was by a process of systematic desensitization. This technique involves two steps, both of which are time-consuming and not always easy to master. First the students were given instructional tapes which taught them how to achieve a state of deep muscular relaxation, then they were encouraged to practise holding this state of ease while they faced up to their anxieties. Those who succeeded in following these instructions found their anxiety was diminished. But equal benefit was derived by a control group of students whose sole treatment was going for a jog while concentrating on pleasantly relaxing thoughts. By working out their tensions in this simple way they lessened their anxiety and scored an impressive improvement in their examination marks. As Richard Driscoll concludes in an article in *The Psychological Review*, jogging is a simpler, quicker way of reducing anxiety than the far more cumbersome technique of desensitization. It can be practised anywhere, requires no therapist or elaborate training, and needs only the barest minimum of equipment.

A further advantage anxious patients derive from taking part in sport is an automatic switching-off from their day-to-day worries. You can't worry about the household bills when you're playing golf and trying to sink a five yard putt. Business problems fade completely from mind when you're concentrating on serving an ace at tennis, and even the most anxious mother finds it impossible to worry about her children when she's in the throes of a fast downhill ski run. (At the time she's

67

probably far too concerned about her own safety to worry about her offsprings' minor coughs and colds and skin rashes!)

People who are beset with cares often try to erase them from their mind. But you can't make the mind a blank. Nature abhors a vacuum and will always fill the brain with thoughts, either pleasant or unpleasant. The only way to chase out the hobgoblins of anxiety is to replace them with the elfins of playfulness and fun. This principle has been taught by gurus of all persuasions for thousands of years. A number have schooled their pupils to switch off from the cares of everyday life by concentrating their gaze on a mandala, a flower, a flickering candle, or a holy relic or icon. Some have trained their disciples to focus their attention by reciting prayers or repeatedly chanting a mantra. Others have employed physical means such as flagellation, pilgrimages, whirling dances, archery training and the maintenance of yoga asanas to concentrate the mind. To people brought up in the Western culture, a more effective way of diverting the mind from non-productive worrying thought is to engage in some form of totally absorbing active pursuit. Some people find relaxation in gardening. Others obtain solace by going on long country walks. (Even the Romans realized the therapeutic value of hiking and had a popular maxim which said 'Walking solves it'.) Fishing is a favourite diversion for many pressurized men. They forget their other cares when they pit their wits against a wily trout. Time stands still as they cast their lines and watch the tell-tale ripples on the water. As a five-thousand-year-old inscription on an Assyrian tablet puts it, 'The gods do not subtract from the allotted span of men's lives the hours spent in fishing.'

Man is by nature a dynamic animal and is never more at peace with the world than when he's engaged in some form of active work, sport or play. And the more active he is, the fitter he becomes both physically and mentally. In the past, a sharp distinction was often drawn between physical and mental health. Children at school were expected to fall into one of two categories: they were either brainy or brawny. It was considered unthinkable that they should excel in both the classroom and the gymnasium. But now it is recognized that mental and physical health are positively correlated. To be psychologically fit and alert, we need to be physically fit and active. The ideal, as Juvenal, the Roman poet, suggested, is to develop a healthy mind in a healthy body (*mens sana in corpore sano*). This can only be done by following a dynamogenic lifestyle.

Research shows that the higher an individual's standard of physical health, the less his risk of suffering mental illness. When Dr Lloyd Appleton of the US Military Academy, West Point, studied the physical fitness and health records of a large group of the Academy's cadets, he discovered that psychological symptoms diminished as fitness increased. He encountered no psychiatric difficulties whatsoever in the very fittest students, but noted that 13 per cent of cadets with the lowest fitness ratings had to be given discharges from the Academy on psychiatric grounds. Active participation in sports and recreational pastimes tends to make people more amiable and sociable. This was confirmed by a study carried out at Aberdeen University, which showed that students who were actively engaged in sport had more stable, less introverted personalities than those who pursued a more sedentary way of life. Their additional amiability and inward calm may result from the greater opportunity they have for abreaction and the release of emotional tension. There would almost certainly be less juvenile delinquency if children were encouraged to be more active and give vent to their natural high spirits in play rather than through acts of vandalism. This was the opinion of the Wolfenden Committee set up by the Central Council of Physical Recreation to investigate the sporting and recreational needs of the British people. In its report *Sport and the Community* the Committee concluded, 'If more young people had opportunities for playing games fewer of them would develop criminal habits.'

People who adopt a more vital way of life can expect to enjoy an automatic decrease in their tensions and anxieties. Without any great effort on their part they will acquire greater equanimity, become more sociable and be less prone to psychosomatic ailments. Those who suffer high levels of tension and stress at present can derive immediate benefit by adopting the following habits which are an intrinsic part of the dynamogenic lifestyle and offer a rapid way of dispelling tension, anxiety and fear:

● *When your way ahead is clear, act, don't procrastinate.* As was pointed out in the previous chapter, timid people often make thinking a substitute for doing. So long as they are busy *planning* their next move, they have a perfect excuse for not *taking* it. They avoid putting a foot wrong by never putting a foot forward. But they miss the bus of life simply because they lack the courage to jump aboard. They watch it carefully as it appears in sight, and peer at it wistfully as it cruises away, but never summon up the initiative to step on board. 'Look before you leap' is their constant watchword, not 'He who hesitates is lost.' So they spend their lives as perpetual voyeurs, always looking at the goodies in the shop window, but never leaping in to make a longed-for purchase. Problems can rarely be solved by sitting down and worrying about them. Generally they are best overcome by taking some course of remedial action. However great the dilemma that faces you, it can normally be surmounted in a series of simple stages. All that is necessary is to plan the stages and make the initial move. Remember that even the most arduous expedition of a thousand miles starts with a single step.

And don't imagine that the journey is made the moment you've chosen your ultimate destination. Aims and ambitions are useless unless they are translated into action. The road to everyone's hell is paved with good intentions. It is only by living out our dreams that we give them substance. As psychologist William James said at the beginning of the century, 'No matter how full a reservoir of maxims one may possess, and no matter how good one's sentiments may be, if one has not taken advantage of every concrete opportunity to *act*, one's character may remain entirely unaffected for the better.'

When Friedrich Nietzsche began to commit his philosophies to paper he was convinced that man's driving force should be the 'will to truth at all costs'. Later he discovered that the pursuit of truth alone was not enough. Man's major motivation, he decided, must be the 'will to live'. Our days are too short to be spent in passive contemplation. They are meant for vigorous and lusty participation. As he wrote in *The Birth of Tragedy*, 'Down with thought – long live life.' People who adopt the dynamogenic lifestyle will be rewarded by a diminution in their anxieties and a marked increase in their happiness.

● *Live in the present.* Pleasure is of the moment, anxiety is invariably of the future or the past. When our mind is preoccupied with worry, it is rarely concerned with contemporary problems which are open to solution, but is far more likely to be engaged in an unproductive review of the missed opportunities, mistakes and failures of the past, or a hypothetical consideration of the difficulties and disasters which could arise in the future. But the only time we can act is now. Nothing we do can alter one syllable of recorded time. If we have behaved unwisely in the past, all we can do to make amends is to learn from our mistakes and behave more sensibly today. Chronic self-denigration and remorse are corrosive sentiments. As Aldous Huxley wrote in *Brave New World*, 'Rolling in the muck is not the best way of getting clean.' In the same way it is inadvisable to invest too much psychic energy in non-productive anxiety about the future. As the Bible says, 'Take therefore no thought for the morrow: for the morrow shall take thought for the things of itself. Sufficient unto the day is the evil thereof.' In any case, why concern yourself with events which, in all probability, will never happen? Anxiety only has a point if it leads to purposeful activity in the here and now. People of an anxious disposition would find their worries decimated if they refused to carry the burden of yesterday's mistakes and tomorrow's troubles, and cultivated instead the art of living for today.

This may appear too much a hedonist's charter for some to accept. We have been schooled to deny the pleasures of the flesh in return for rewards which will be heaped upon us in the great beyond. Generations of political reformers have given up present satisfaction in order to pave the way for a distant Utopia. The promise has always been jam tomorrow, but never jam today. But we are ephemeral creatures. We have only one time to live, and that is *now*. To be fulfilled, our lives must be filled to the full. To achieve our maximum potential, we must put aside the petty anxieties which paralyse our will to act, and allow ourselves the freedom to grow, create, experiment and explore. We must constantly remind ourselves of the Latin maxim *Carpe diem* (Reap the day).

This precept, although sadly understated in Judaeo-Christian teaching, is an inherent part of Zen Buddhism. Zen teaches its followers to concentrate simply and exclusively on the present. When they eat they are enjoined to focus their attention solely on the act of eating and not to dissipate their energies thinking about the weather, their work, or the rising cost of living. Similarly, when they work they are advised to concentrate totally on the job in hand, and not divert their attention by planning their next meal or reorganizing the household budget. In this way, they increase their efficiency and maximize their enjoyment of every act they perform. This was confirmed by the work of Abraham Maslow, one of the founders of the school of humanistic psychology, who noted that whenever people enjoyed moments of ecstasy, which he described as 'peak experiences', they were totally absorbed in the 'here and now'. This, he found, was equally true of moments of great creativity. As he wrote, 'This ability to become "lost in the present" seems to be a *sine qua non* for creativeness of any kind.'

The prophet Mohammed shared the same doctrine, and encouraged his disciples to live in the tangible present rather than in the chimerical future. This was one of the things that attracted heavy-weight boxer Mohammed Ali to the Muslim faith. For years he'd been fobbed off with the white man's promise of 'pie in the sky when you die by-and-by'. Then came the far more appealing advice of the Black Muslim preachers, calling upon the faithful to fulfil their desires 'down on the ground while you're still around'. 'Here and now', they said, is the only conceivable time and place for things to happen.

If we are to conquer our troublesome fears, we must bury the demons of the past and refuse to conjure up the hobgoblins of the future. We must live each day as if it were our last on earth. As the legendary blind writer Helen Keller said, 'Use your eyes as if tomorrow you would be stricken blind; hear the music of voices, the song of a bird, as if you would be stricken deaf tomorrow. Touch each object as if tomorrow your tactile sense would fail. Smell the perfume of flowers, taste with relish each morsel, as if tomorrow you could never smell and taste again.' In this way, through a total absorption in the trivial activities of daily life, we can escape anxiety and find contentment.

● *Act spontaneously.* Children are born with the gift of acting in a natural, free and unpremeditated fashion. As we grow older we lose this delightful freshness and spontaneity. We acquire social inhibitions and restraints which make us censor our instinctive responses. Often we suppress our natural desire to act by a prolonged analysis of the possible consequences. Like the proverbial centipede we become paralysed when we stop to decide which leg to move first. Your impulsive wish may be to throw an impromptu bottle party, but if you're not careful this delightful idea will be vetoed by the gloomy cautioning of your conscious mind. Most of your friends will have other engagements and give you the brush-off. They'll think it strange if they're asked to bring their own liquor. Anyway, what about food? You'll never get even a snack meal together in the limited time available. Besides, it's not your turn to give a party. And in any case, what will the neighbours say if you go ahead with this crazy idea? There are always a hundred excuses to sanction idleness and lack of adventure. Maybe you have a sudden urge to go away for the weekened and visit friends. Then your kill-joy conscience starts to work. It's a long journey. Maybe the hotels will be fully booked. What if your friends have other plans and don't really want to see you? And what about the work that needs to be done in the garden? So you let the wet blanket of hypercritical concerns kill the flames of spontaneous desire. To overcome this block it's sometimes necessary to act first and think afterwards. To restore a measure of spontaneity in our lives we should whenever possible listen to the inner promptings of the body and sleep when we're tired, eat when we're hungry, weep when we're sad, laugh when we're happy and make love whenever we feel the sudden promptings of erotic desire. In this way our actions will be natural, free and unselfconscious.

● *Direct your thoughts outwards; don't be self-possessed or morbidly introspective.* Anxiety is largely self-induced. Anyone can become a hypochondriac if he pays sufficient attention to the inner workings of his body. If you put aside this book for a few moments and carefully monitor the sensations emanating from inside your body you could no doubt list ten or more potentially alarming symptoms. That slight stiffness in your neck might be the sign of arthritis. That twinge of indigestion could be the start of an ulcer. If you worry about these possibilities your heart will beat a little faster. For safety's sake you check your pulse rate. Maybe it's pounding away at 82 beats a minute. Isn't the normal rate only 72? You make a second count and this time you detect a distinct skipped beat. Is this the sign of an impending heart attack? You slump in the chair and immediately notice that you're panting heavily. You see the colour draining from your skin. Anxiety holds you in a vice-like grip. You feel a stab of tension pain across your chest. This confirms your worst fears. The telltale combination of pallor, laboured breathing, chest pain and a fluttering pulse can mean only one thing: you're about to have a heart attack.

This account may seem fanciful, but many people do in fact make themselves ill by paying excessive attention to their bodies. Doctors estimate that 10 to 30 per cent of the population are the victims of hypochondriasis. For some this is a crippling malaise – men like the multi-millionaire Howard Hughes whose whole life was taken over by a paranoid concern to avoid eating contaminated food or coming into contact with pathogenic germs; or the financier John D. Rockefeller who was so fearful of being smitten by sudden illness that he always travelled with a supply of oxygen and had fully-equipped private hospitals installed in every one of his homes.

The answer to the problem of hypochondriasis lies in exchanging an obsessive interest with the self for a passionate involvement in the world at large. This was the salvation of the poet Elizabeth Browning, who was a self-made invalid for the first forty years of her life. As a young girl she had suffered a minor spinal injury and this she magnified into a major disability which gave her a valid excuse for leading the life of a recluse and escaping the demands of her tyrannical father. Most of her days she spent propped up on a couch. Because of her frailty, visitors to her sickroom were barred, including William Wordsworth who admired her poetry and several times expressed a keen desire to meet her. Then she met the spirited Robert Browning who metaphorically swept her off her feet, but literally placed her feet firmly on the ground. Through him she began to take an interest in the outside world. Instead of being incarcerated in her sick room, she travelled extensively throughout Europe. Instead of refusing to receive guests in the interests of her health, she enjoyed the stimulus of meeting many of the literary giants of the age – Tennyson, George Sand, Kingsley and Ruskin. Instead of protecting her body from the slightest stress or strain she took up the arduous sport of mountain-climbing. Instead of living only for herself, Elizabeth Browning gave herself unstintingly to her husband, and she bore him a son at the age of forty-three. So she lost her morbid preoccupation with her personal problems and as a consequence discovered the rich rewards of an outward-looking, dynamogenic lifestyle.

The same is true of people who are constantly

worried about their personal problems. They fret about their jobs. Are they going to be overworked when they take the new job that's been offered them? Will they find themselves redundant when the proposed merger takes place? They worry about their appearance. Are they looking old? Are they too fat/thin/stooped/pale/wrinkled/grey? They're anxious about their homes. Should they increase their insurance? Is it time to consider moving to a smaller house with a more easily maintained garden? They worry too about the impression they make on their friends. Are they as popular as they should be? Do people think they're old-fashioned? Anxieties like these mount whenever people can see no further than the problems of their own small world. Tensions lessen the moment we look outside ourselves and take a lively interest in the welfare of others. You're unlikely to sit and mope about your ingrowing toenail if you're going out and helping a neighbour who's recently lost a leg in a car crash. And while you're actively helping the homeless in the neighbourhood, you're less prone to worry about the few tiles missing from the roof of your own comfortable home. In fact, there's nothing like an active interest in other people's problems to overcome a pathological obsession with one's own.

Some years ago Carl Jung, the eminent Swiss psychologist, drew a sharp distinction between introversion and extroversion. He noted that extroverts, like Benvenuto Cellini, Samuel Pepys, Donald Duck and Mr Punch, were outward-looking, gregarious, lively and adventurous people, whereas introverts like Hamlet, Faust and Kant were more passive, reserved, introspective and cerebral. He also found that symptoms of anxiety were considerably more common among introverts than among extroverts. This has since been confirmed by numerous personality studies which suggest that anxiety can be lessened by adopting a more active, outward-looking approach to life.

For three years research workers at Leeds University studied the fate of eighty-three patients attending the University's Department of Psychiatry. Half were suffering from anxiety states, the remainder from miscellaneous psychoneurotic disorders such as hypochondriasis, depression, impotence and hysterical conversion symptoms. All were judged to be in need of expert psychotherapy, which for one reason or another they failed to receive. Nevertheless, even without the assistance of skilled medical treatment, it was found that people who had a satisfying job and a wide variety of outside interests showed a remarkably high rate of spontaneous recovery. Interviews revealed that 67 per cent of the patients who recovered completely had extraneous interests in such things as political organizations, trade unions and clubs, whereas these group affiliations were enjoyed by only 23 per cent of the patients who showed only partial improvement and by none of the subjects who showed no tendency whatsoever to natural recovery. As the research team reported, the outstanding characteristic of these long-term psychiatric casualties and chronic worriers was that they 'all tended to live in small isolated worlds, with their thoughts and activities rarely directed beyond themselves.'

● *Cultivate a wide range of interests.* If you're a member of a church choir, actively engaged in singing the Hallelujah Chorus, you're unlikely to be worrying about your children's abysmal record at school. If at the weekend you're sailing a dinghy through heavy seas, you've no time to think about the problem of raising money to finance your coming holiday. Anxiety invariably arises in times of idleness. We have no time to worry if we keep our bodies and minds occupied with healthy pursuits.

Charles Darwin was a chronic worrier, but found that he could escape his problems by playing billiards. To help him unwind he had a table installed in Down House, his delightful home in the Kent countryside, during the year he completed work on *The Origin of Species*. 'I find it does me a deal of good,' he wrote to a friend, 'and drives the horrid species out of my head.' British television personality Hughie Green finds solace by playing with his model railway. 'I find that after a hard day I can switch on the trains and switch off the worries,' he reports. Lord Nuffield, the car magnate, relaxed by toying with bits and pieces of machinery. 'When I can't sleep at night, I get up and use my hands,' he said. 'I have to be fixing something, building something. It gives me release; gets rid of tensions.'

Taking part in risk activities is a particularly effective way of dispelling anxieties. The trivial problems of day-to-day living disappear from your mind when you're making a free-fall parachute descent, or shooting the rapids in a raft. At moments like these you've got to concentrate on the task in hand. These adrenalin-releasing activities can also produce a feeling of euphoria, akin to the 'high' that comes from taking psychedelic drugs. According to a study made by Dr Sol Roy Rosenthal, Professor of Preventive Medicine at the University of Illinois, 97 per cent of athletes find that they get a greater feeling of elation, well-being and physical invigoration when taking part in risk activities such as mountain-climbing, skiing, horseback riding and gliding, than when they participate in less dangerous sports such as golf, jogging and calisthenics. This has been the experience of the members of Oxford University's Dangerous Sports Club, who have travelled the world in search of thrills. During the two years of the club's existence members have skateboarded in front of the free-running bulls of Pamplona, leapt off the summit of Mount Kilimanjaro in hang-gliders, and sought to emulate the vine-jumping feats of the natives of New Guinea by jumping off the Clifton Suspension Bridge, poised 250 feet above the Avon Gorge, with only a thin elasticated cord strapped to their backs to save them from certain death. As their leader David Kirk explains, 'We do these stunts to try and get away from the boredom of plastic pressurized everyday living. Most people may think we are mad. We think they are insane to endure such humdrum lives. The instant you jump out into thin air from a bridge or mountain is the moment you experience 100 per cent awareness of life. In that moment all the everyday pressures become irrelevant, and it doesn't matter whether your car needs washing or your mortgage payments are not up to date.'

People who adopt the dynamogenic programme outlined in this book will find that their lives will become infinitely more rich and exciting, and far less ridden with anxieties and fears – without the need to take perilous leaps off suspension bridges and mountain tops! If we are to regain our equanimity, we must lead more exuberant, vital lives. If we fail to do so, we could all too easily exchange our cushioned chambers for anxiety-ridden padded cells.

5

The Drugless Cure For Rheumatism

Rheumatism is another of the crippling by-products of hypokinetic living. Statistics show that this is now one of the major problems of the Western world. Each year in Britain eight million people go to their doctors for help with rheumatic complaints, which give rise to a loss of over thirty million working days. In America it is believed that over twelve million people suffer from arthritis alone, and recent estimates suggest that the rheumatic diseases are now costing the US economy over one billion dollars in lost production.

Why this appalling toll of ill health? Why should nations with such outstandingly high standards of medical care endure so much chronic invalidism? Some people look for an explanation in the food we eat or in the chemical pollution of the water we drink. But in truth the answer does not lie in our devitalized diet, but in our devitalized lives. The vast majority of people who suffer rheumatic pain and disability today do so because their lives provide too little movement to preserve either the strength of their muscles or the suppleness of their joints.

Young farmers often express surprise that they should suffer so much more rheumatic pain than their elderly fathers, who led a much tougher life. But this is easily explained. A century ago a farmer tilled his fields walking behind a horse-drawn plough. Every one of the thousands of steps he took during the course of his working day strengthened the powerful muscles of his back and loosened the joints of his pelvis and spine. He had little chance then of developing a weak or stiff back. Now he does the same job riding on a tractor – a physically undemanding task that allows his joints and muscles to grow stiff and weak. He also suffers the postural strain of sitting for hours on end in a slumped position. (Recent ergonomic studies show that this strain is often aggravated because many tractor seats vibrate at frequencies of about 3½ cycles per second, which is dangerously near 4 cycles per second – the natural frequency of the lumbar spine. This means that resonance can occur, with the spine bouncing up and down like a ping-pong ball in a jet of water.)

In the same way the modern housewife may suffer more fibrositic pain than her grandmother, even though her home is now equipped with every conceivable labour-saving gadget. The reason is that her daily routine deprives her of much opportunity to bend, twist, stretch and turn, while not sparing her the fatiguing postural strain of standing over sinks, work-tops and ironing boards. In fact she is now more immobilized than ever before. For hours on end she stands or sits in positions of postural strain. Instead of walking to the shops, she now travels by car. Instead of having her groceries delivered to the door, she is forced to drag her purchases round the supermarket, manhandle them into the boot of her car and then unload them into the house. This involves far more tension and strain for her shoulder muscles. When she does the family laundry, she doesn't wash the clothes by hand each day as her grandmother did, scrubbing them maybe on an old-fashioned washboard, rinsing them in a tub of clean water, then hanging them on an outside line to dry. Instead she stock-piles the week's dirty linen so that she can make proper economic use of the launderette or washing machine. She forgoes the vigorous exercise of scrubbing the clothes clean in a tub of water or a stream, and replaces it with the tension of lifting heavy piles of clothing into a washing machine. In exchange for the healthy exercise of stretching up to peg a series of items of clothing on an outside washing line, she substitutes the strain of lifting a heap of sodden linen into a spin dryer. Then, to add to her washing day tensions and postural strains, instead of doing her ironing each day, a few minutes at a time, she's now prepared to iron for several hours at a stretch to get the chore completed. This particular folly would not have been possible before the advent of the electric iron, for flat irons had to be heated every few minutes over an open fire, which made it impossible to subject the back to the postural strain of non-stop ironing.

Rheumatism is just as much a product of twentieth-century living as water beds, midnight movies and takeaway fried chicken. Each of the three most common forms of rheumatism – fibrositis, backache and degenerative arthritis – have strong causative links with our modern sedentary way of life. All three will become more common unless we halt our slide into an increasingly pampered, indolent lifestyle.

Consider first the problem of fibrositis or muscular rheumatism. Muscles form about 42 per cent of the weight of the average male, and 36 per cent of the weight of the average female, and are probably responsible for more than 90 per cent of rheumatic pain. All the most painful medical conditions – gall-stones, renal colic, appendicitis, childbirth and heart attacks – are associated with internal muscle spasm. Labour pains are caused almost entirely by the sustained contraction of the uterine muscles and these pangs can be greatly lessened, as was shown convincingly by Dr Grantly Dick Read, the pioneer of Natural Childbirth Training, if mothers are taught to relax their pelvic muscles between uterine contractions. Even eating pounds of sour apples wouldn't have such disastrous consequences if it didn't make the muscles of the intestines knot up like strands of convoluted spaghetti.

Similar pains arise in the body's limb muscles. Use them as Nature intended and they won't utter a word of complaint. Employ them under conditions of sustained tension and they'll soon give rise to fibrositic pain. A muscle like the biceps in the arm can be contracted and

83

relaxed a thousand times during the course of a game of tennis without producing any discomfort whatsoever, but if it is held in sustained contraction for a minute or more it soon begins to ache. This you can easily prove by a simple experiment. Keeping an eye on your watch, bend and straighten your arm for a minute. You will be able to achieve this easily and with no sense of strain. Now flex your arm to a right angle and tense your biceps as tightly as you can, if necessary by gripping your wrist with your opposite hand and firmly resisting any further bending of the arm. This will normally produce a pronounced ache in the arm within thirty to sixty seconds. This proves, if proof is necessary, that our muscles were intended to be used in a relaxed cycle of intermittent work and rest, rather than held on sustained tension.

Even the strongest man in the world would experience pain in his forearm if he tried to maintain his maximum grip for two or three minutes. No wonder then that school children sitting exams develop forearm pain when they nervously grip their pens for three hours at a stretch, and housewives experience fibrositic pain in their shoulders after submitting their muscles to the constant strain of carrying a ten-pound bag of shopping. A large proportion of our activities today involve the holding of similarly tense and static postures. As job specialization increases these poses become more limited and cramped. A dentist will spend a working lifetime in a frozen posture more suited to a gnarled oak tree than a living, freely moving human being. For years their bodies cope with this unnaturally stunted lifestyle, and then the rheumatic pains begin. The necks which have been bent like shepherds' crooks, peering at gingivous gums and carious canines, suddenly become seized with muscular spasms. The left hands, which for years have clasped reamers, scaler curettes and peridontal probes, finally become the seat of muscle cramps and painful tendons. And the backs, which have been bent like broken matchsticks over a gaggle of dental patients, eventually succumb to postural fatigue and severe lumbago.

Muscles were never meant to be used in a state of prolonged tension. A working muscle needs a plentiful supply of blood to supply the actively contracting muscle fibres with oxygen and remove the waste products of muscle metabolism. When they are working vigorously muscles may need ten times as much blood as they receive when they are at rest. This they cannot possibly obtain while they are contracting, for when muscles contract they clamp down on the intramuscular blood vessels and so reduce the circulatory flow. It is only during the phase of relaxation that muscles can be adequately replenished with blood. For this reason it is essential that periods of activity should always be alternated with periods of rest. If muscles are held in a state of prolonged tension they suffer a mounting accumulation of metabolic waste products and an increasing shortage of oxygen. This produces both fatigue and pain. To prevent this happening, muscles must be used like piston engines, with an explosive burst of energy followed by a slow recovery stroke.

The large postural muscles of the neck, shoulders, back and pelvis in particular need to be given regular periods of rest. It is significant in this respect to note that all the natural bodily movements – walking, running, swimming, dancing – involve a rhythmical cycle of alternate phases of work and rest. Using the body in this way is sensually pleasing and produces little discomfort or unhealthy fatigue. Contrast this with the lethargy and pain that comes from tense, 'civilized' activities such as driving a car, carrying heavy shopping, bending over an office desk or sitting slumped in front of a TV set. If we have to perform these chores, we must see that they are relieved by regular periods of activity. No typist should be expected to bend over her typewriter for more than an hour at a stretch. After this time she should be encouraged to get up from her desk and engage in some other form of activity, such as filing, sorting through the mail, or photocopying. If cellists are going to spend hours a day straddling their ungainly instruments, they must be trained to take up pursuits like swimming, skipping or running, which provide an antidote for their occupational strain. Weekend gardeners must acquire the habit of varying their chores so that they don't spend an entire morning bending over a vegetable plot, but instead ring the changes between reaching up and clipping a length of hedge, kneeling down to thin out some seedlings, twisting over to repair a garden fence and then stretching up to tie a straggling piece of clematis. This will keep the body on the move and help to prevent the onset of postural strain.

This same principle must also be employed in industry. Wherever possible job rotation schemes should be introduced so that factory workers can have the mental stimulus and physical respite of frequent changes of activity. At regular periods during the day production line workers should be encouraged to stand back from the assembly line and take part in a short series of gymnastic exercises. Five minute keep-fit classes can be organized during coffee breaks to stimulate the circulation and stretch out tense muscle groups. Experience in several East European countries has proved the value of these brief sessions of 'break gymnastics'. An alternative method of tension release has been employed in at least one factory in Japan, where girls engaged on the intricate task of assembling transistorized equipment are advised to step back from their work at regular intervals to give their bodies and limbs a delicious overall stretch. These thirty-second 'yawning sessions' have been found to improve production and lessen tension and fatigue.

Everyone engaged in specialized work involving the maintenance of static postures – musicians, machine operators, draughtsmen, typists, housewives and desk-bound executives – should acquire the habit of injecting as much movement as posssible into their day's routine.

Whenever possible, they should shift their weight from side to side, change hands, alter their pose, stretch, bend, laugh, gesticulate, sing, stride over to the coffee dispenser and run up and down stairs. Even performing a dozen half-knee bends on every visit to the toilet would help prevent the early onset of postural strain and muscular fatigue.

It is noticeable that in recent years there has been a marked shift in the incidence of occupational complaints. Two or three centuries ago workers tended to suffer because they subjected their bodies to unaccustomed over-use. At the start of every shooting season many gillies in Scotland would suffer from 'gamekeeper's knee' – a painful inflammation at the back of the knee caused by repeatedly lifting the legs to clamber over bracken, gorse and heather. Prior to the Industrial Revolution, inexperienced weavers were prone to succumb to 'weaver's bottom' – an uncomfortable inflammation of the tissues protecting the bony haunches of the pelvis. This arose because they were constantly sliding up and down their bench seats to reach the extremities of their looms. (It also explains Shakespeare's choice of the name 'Bottom the Weaver' for his comic character in *A Midsummer Night's Dream* – a play on words which would have been readily appreciated by seventeenth-century audiences.) Nowadays, few occupational maladies arise from physical over-use. If a gamekeeper suffers pain in his leg today, it's most likely to arise from the postural strain of keeping his right foot constantly poised on the accelerator of his Land Rover, and if a modern textile operator gets a painful rump it won't be the result of frantically sliding up and down his bench but from the postural strain of standing still watching the dials of his electronically controlled power loom. Our twentieth-century occupational hazards are those primarily of tense inactivity, like writer's cramp, typist's neck and pilot's back. The answer to these problems is activity rather than rest. Just as the easiest way to get rid of nocturnal leg cramps is to get out of bed and walk about, so the quickest way to cure fibrositic muscle spasms is to subject the offending muscles to vigorous use. A tense neck will not lose its stiffness by being encased in an orthopaedic collar, nor will a painful, rigid back be restored to full mobility if it is incarcerated in a spinal jacket.

Muscles like to be used, both in sickness and in health. The larger muscles of the body, like the biceps and hamstrings, can withstand a pull of several hundred pounds before they show any sign of injury. To tear the calf muscle of a healthy middle-aged man, for example, it is necessary to exert a sudden jerk of something in the region of 400 kilos (900 lb). Forces of this nature generally arise only when we make a sudden, unexpected movement. A tennis player is wrongly footed, tries to change direction, and feels a sudden stab of pain in his calf as if he's been shot by a gun. At this moment he will no doubt have torn several fibres in his calf muscle. As long as the muscle is not totally ruptured, this injury will heal completely within a matter of two or three weeks, *providing the leg continues to be used*. But if the leg is immobilized, or cossetted by a protective limp, the pain and disability may persist for months on end. And if adhesions form as a result of disuse, the muscle may become the site of repeated injury. This happened frequently in the past, when it was customary to immobilize damaged muscles for four to six weeks in either a plaster cast or a cocoon of adhesive bandages. This gave rise to the adage, frequently repeated by athletic coaches, 'Once a strain always a strain.' But there should be no tendency to chronic weakness providing the injured muscles continue to be used while they're healing. The reason for this is simple. Whenever muscle fibres are torn or severely over-stretched, tiny blood vessels are damaged. This leads to a degree of intramuscular bleeding, and the release of blood cells, called fibroblasts, which are responsible for the production of new fibrous tissue and the healing of the damaged muscle cells. The distribution and arrangement of these strands of fibrous tissue is entirely dependent on the mechanical forces acting on the muscle. If the muscle is subjected to regular use while it is healing, the reparative tissue can only be deposited in an orderly fashion along the line of muscle pull. But if the muscle is immobilized, or allowed to remain idle, the network of fibrous tissue tends to be deposited in a haphazard fashion, forming adhesive links between adjacent bunches of muscle fibres. This gives rise to a painful limitation of movement when full activity is resumed. To prevent this happening, the muscle should be used as normally as possible while healing takes place.

The only recommended treatment for a muscle injury is the immediate application of cold water packs for ten minutes, followed by the quickest possible return to full activity. The reason for the application of cold water is to limit the extent of intra-muscular bleeding. On no account should heat be applied to a recently damaged muscle until the risk of bleeding is over. This may take up to forty-eight hours. (The old idea of applying heat to damaged muscles to 'draw out the bruise' merely increased the extent of intra-muscular bleeding.) When treated with cold water packs, muscle injuries heal both rapidly and well. A short while ago an international sprinter tore the muscles of his thigh during a race meeting. A generation ago he might have been swathed in bandages and put to bed. Instead, he was given the immediate task of hobbling round the track until he could jog without an appreciable limp. The next day he was asked to repeat this exercise and then perform a few short sprints at three-quarters of his normal top speed. After three days he was able to run at full speed. Five days later he was fit enough to compete in a race and celebrated his recovery by recording his fastest-ever time, even though his leg at the time was bruised from buttock to knee! Exercise is demonstrably the ideal tonic for healthy muscles, and also the finest natural restorative for muscles that are weak, stiff, tired, tense or torn.

Movement is also the finest prophylactic against backache. Insurance companies in Britain have bemoaned the fact that since the 'discovery' of the slipped disc the invalidism caused by spinal aches and pains has soared. A generation ago most back pains were attributed to lumbago, and treated by heat and movement. Now they are more commonly ascribed to herniations or tears of the intervertebral discs, and treated by analgesic pills and prolonged bed rest. This has increased the invalidism. The spinal column is a marvel of engineering skill but it needs to be kept in constant use to preserve its health. Like a veteran motor car, or an ancient piece of farm machinery, it functions best when it's maintained in regular use, not when it's wrapped in protective covers. Every one of its component parts deteriorates if they are allowed to remain idle. The back muscles need daily exercise to maintain their tone. Spinal joints need to be constantly flexed to retain their suppleness. Intervertebral discs rely on regular movement to ensure their proper nourishment, and the spinal ligaments require constant stretching to preserve their elasticity. It's a mistake to think of the spinal column as a delicate rod which needs to be protected from bending strains and torsional stresses. It becomes weak only when it's allowed to suffer the atrophy of disuse. A healthy, active spine can with impunity lift weights of several hundred pounds and perform cartwheels, somersaults and yoga *asanas* without the slightest strain.

Naturally, like every other part of the body, the spine will be the site of occasional pain. But this is seldom an occasion for alarm, and rarely a cause for medical treatment. Just as the average bout of indigestion will disappear without going to bed or taking antacid powders, so the majority of episodes of lumbago will clear up spontaneously without the need for wearing spinal jackets, rubbing in counter-irritant creams or taking muscle relaxant drugs. Surveys show that most cases of backache recover without medical treatment – 75 per cent within a week, 98 per cent within a month. But despite this welcome tendency of the body to heal itself, the world is still populated with millions of people suffering from chronic backache. This is almost certainly the greatest single cause of avoidable suffering and invalidism. The great tragedy is that most individuals plagued with persistent back pains are not suffering from incurable orthopaedic maladies such as rheumatoid arthritis, but from simple mechanical problems which could easily be remedied, like stiff joints, contracted ligaments and tense muscles. The great bulk of these disorders could be avoided by adopting the dynamogenic programme outlined in this book.

The commonest causes of backache are tension, lack of exercise and postural strain. These are all by-products of our sedentary way of life. Tests carried out at the Institute for Physical Medicine and Rehabilitation at New York University have shown that fully 80 per cent of backache is due to muscular tension or weakness. These deficiencies can be overcome by carrying out the mobility exercises shown on pages 273–6 and the muscle-strengthening exercises outlined on pages 277–82.

Hypokinesis affects the back in many subtle ways. As a result primarily of lack of exercise we overeat and become obese. This immediately disturbs the normal mechanics of the spine. Since we carry most of our excess weight on the abdomen, like pregnant penguins, it becomes necessary to arch the back to keep the centre of gravity of our bodies over our feet. This results in constant postural strain on the lumbar area of our spines. Insufficient exercise also leads to weakness of the muscles of the belly and back. This predisposes the spine to further strain by removing its protective muscular corset. Weakening of the muscles of the buttocks and abdomen also permits the spine to sink into a more pronounced hollow, which leads to additional postural strain. Disuse also decreases the suppleness of the muscles of the back which makes them more prone to strain. At this point the body, recognizing the increasing vulnerability of the spine, makes an attempt to increase its defences by maintaining a level of guarding muscle tension. If prolonged this is itself a cause of pain and fatigue, particularly since the back muscles are likely to be under a high degree of tension already, as a result of occupational strains and the unresolved stresses of modern life. In time, this state of habitual tension gives way to permanent shortening of the muscle fibres, for nature abhors waste and can see no point in maintaining muscles in a state of active contraction when it can achieve the same result by holding them in a state of fixed and effortless contraction. So the back gets progressively stiffer and more prone to damage. This results in more pain, which leads to further protective muscle spasm and an increasing tendency to protect the back by inhibiting all forms of potentially painful movement. So the vicious cycle develops, as shown in the diagram below.

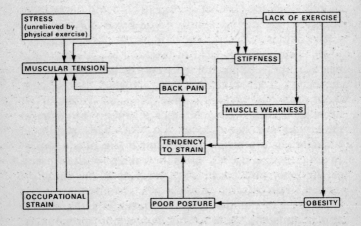

The simplest way to break this harmful sequence of events is to regain the full mobility of the back. This is the secret of the osteopath's success in treating cases of chronic back pain. There is no mystery about spinal manipulation. Its function is not to replace slipped discs or correct spinal alignment, but to restore movement. In essence, it is little more than an accurately directed form of assisted exercise. And it works even in relatively unskilled hands. One physician took up manipulation when he grew dissatisfied with the orthodox treatment of back pain and was soon delighted with his results. As he reported in the medical press, 'There are very few cases of backache with or without sciatic pain that cannot be cured by manipulation or traction (stretching).' Another doctor made a three-year study of the subject and concluded, 'Manipulation and accurate manual methods have a great and urgent part to play in general practice.' On the basis of his experience he told his colleagues, 'Any doctor who follows this suggested line of treatment would have the satisfaction of curing most of his sufferers from "rheumatism" and "fibrositis".'

But many cases of backache can be cured without medical or osteopathic treatment by pursuing the exercises described on pages 273–6 or by taking up rhythmical activities such as dancing, swimming or jogging. A short while ago the General Council and Register of Osteopaths drew attention to the fact that every day in Britain 50,000 men and women were away from work because of backache. 'Most of this could be avoided,' their spokesman said, 'if sedentary workers with bad backs would give up long business lunches, quit their television sets in the evening and take a short jog.' One of the great values of a daily walk or jog is that it helps maintain the flexibility of the spine. Every time we take a step forward the pelvis performs a number of gentle gyrations, the hips rise and fall, and the buttocks rotate forwards and backwards. When we break into a trot the amplitude of these movements increases. During the course of a fifteen-minute jog the joints of the spine and pelvis receive about 2,500 of these gentle stretching movements which loosen the spinal joints and tone the muscles of the pelvis, back and abdomen. The same occurs during swimming or dancing. By performing these activities regularly everyone can be his own osteopath, and maintain the health of his own spine.

It is interesting to note in this respect that several folk cures for rheumatism demand a high degree of physical mobility. This is probably the main basis for their curative powers.

In Britain there is an ancient Cornish remedy that evokes the protective power of a magic circle. Outside the quaintly named village of Lanyon Quoit there is a doughnut-shaped boulder called the Men-a-Tol. Local custom holds that people will be cured of their backache if they manage to crawl through the stone's central hole without touching its sides. The original reason for observing this practice was to escape from the painful clutches of the devil, who couldn't pass through a magic circle. Faith probably played a part in the cure, but no doubt considerable benefit was also derived from the gymnastic feat of repeatedly trying to wriggle through the gap in the stone without touching its sides. A similar remedy exists in Germany where many sufferers from lumbago make a pilgrimage to St Michael's Church in Bamberg, where they endeavour to clamber through the tiny gap in the tomb of Bishop Otto of Pommern, who died in 1139 and is said to have possessed the gift of healing, and gave instructions that when he died he was to be buried in such a way that sufferers from lumbago and similar maladies could continue to keep in close contact with him. So a gap was left in his sarcophagus which was constructed rather like a knee-hole desk. Many victims of chronic back pain claim to find relief by making the journey to Bamberg and squirming through the sacred gap in Otto's tomb. But then they would probably have derived equal benefit if they had stayed at home and performed a set of suitable exercises. This is certainly the experience of firms who have offered their employees classes in back-stretching exercises to reduce the toll of spinal injuries.

Some years ago the management of the Owens-Illinois Glass Company, the world's largest glass manufacturers, grew alarmed at the growth of sickness absenteeism among their employees caused by low back pains. Wishing to reduce this wastage of skilled labour, they invited a doctor trained in physical medicine to investigate the dilemma and take whatever steps he thought necessary to bring it under control. The doctor quickly spotted the root cause of the problem. Large numbers of the firm's employees were developing painful backs from prolonged stooping over their machines during a working day which provided them with little opportunity to bend and stretch their spines. The solution was equally obvious: to find a way to encourage the employees to get more exercise for their backs. To this end foremen were trained to spot incipient signs of backache. The moment workers showed the slightest sign of stiffness as they straightened up from their benches they were invited to step back from the production line and perform a standardized set of exercises to loosen their spines. If this simple first aid treatment failed to bring relief they were sent to the factory clinic where a specially trained physiotherapist mobilized their stiff spinal joints and contracted fibrous tissues with manipulation and stretching exercises. This simple regime of treatment produced immediate benefits. Within fifteen months the firm's toll of absenteeism from low back troubles had fallen to a tenth of its previous level, and directors of the company declared themselves 'astounded and gratified' by the results obtained.

If this policy were generally adopted, the toll of backache could be decimated. Unfortunately, when back sufferers attend hospital they are frequently given exercises which are totally inappropriate for their needs.

Most people injure their backs when they are bending forward, lifting a weight or carrying a heavy piece of furniture. This strains the ligaments at the rear of the spine and results in protective spasm in the back's extensor muscles. Unless full mobility is regained soon after this injury adhesions form, and some of the flexibility of the spine is lost. This makes it difficult to bend forward – a range of movement that is easily lost since we rarely have call to make use of our full range of forward flexion. (Unless you perform daily calisthenic exercises, when did you last bend down to touch your toes?) This problem is aggravated when we're under stress, which tenses up the back muscles and further reduces the flexibility of the spine. This is the dilemma which afflicts most sufferers from chronic low back pain. Through a combination of tension, postural strain and flexion injuries, they develop a spine which is too rigid to bend forward easily. This makes it uncomfortable to stand, painful to slump in a chair, and hazardous to bend forward to pick up weights, or work in a semi-flexed position. What these patients badly need is a course of exercises to restore their spine's full range of forward flexion. What they invariably get when they go to hospital is the direct opposite – a standard series of back extension exercises. This does little to remedy their basic deficiency, and may even aggravate their trouble if their backs are already painfully over-extended. Tests carried out ten years ago at Guy's Hospital, London, showed that 50 per cent of patients with back pain attending the hospital's outpatients clinic were made worse following the usual routine of back extension exercises. Despite the publicity given to this adverse report in the medical press, these ineffectual, potentially harmful exercises are still routinely prescribed at thousands of hospitals throughout the world.

Rheumatism as we experience it today is largely a deficiency disease. Just as a shortage of Vitamin C causes scurvy, so a lack of activity leads to disorders of the body's locomotor system. We need movement just as much as we need food and water. Without it bones soften, muscles weaken and joints decay.

Large numbers of people in the Western world suffer from osteoarthritis, a degenerative disease of the joints which is generally associated with old age, but which often starts to appear from the age of eighteen onwards. This is now so common that by the age of fifty 85 per cent of people have radiological evidence of osteoarthritis in the upper regions of their spine. What is responsible for this widespread joint decay? In the lay mind, and in the opinion of many doctors, osteoarthritis is the result of simple 'wear and tear'. According to this theory, just as the bearings of a motor car engine become roughened from regular use, so the linings of our joints suffer the gradual attrition of daily usage. But this analogy is false. Laboratory investigations have shown that animal joints are extremely resistant to normal wear, but cannot tolerate immobility. Our joints, in fact, are far more liable to rust away than to wear away. Biologists have tested the resilience of animal joints by loading them with weights and fixing them in a machine which moves them rapidly backwards and forwards. After twenty-four hours of this gruelling non-stop test, which simulates the effect of several weeks of normal use, there is no evidence of even microscopic wear in the joint tissues.

This amazing resistance to wear is due to the unique properties of the cartilage which lines the joint surfaces. This has a remarkable ability to absorb shocks and offers so little frictional resistance to movement that it is 50 per cent smoother than a skate moving across a sheet of polished ice, and ten times more slippery than the most efficient oil-lubricated engine bearing. Problems arise only when joints are fixed and prevented from moving.

Experiments on dogs, conducted at the University of Texas, have clearly shown the damaging effect of immobility. For varying lengths of time the left knees of these dogs were fixed in a semi-flexed position which did not

97

prevent them from running about. All their other joints were left free, and remained in a healthy state throughout the course of the experiment. But the restricted knee joints quickly showed signs of deterioration. After a fortnight's disuse, there was a noticeable encroachment of fatty connective tissue within the immobilized joints. Dense adhesions had also begun to form between their opposing joint surfaces. After forty-five days it was possible to detect degeneration in the articular cartilage lining the joint sufaces. This was followed a fortnight later by the formation of new bone beneath the areas of eroded cartilage. In other words, less than two months' inactivity had produced degenerative changes in the articular cartilage and underlying bone which were, as the research workers observed, 'similar to the changes observed clinically in ageing joints and in joints with osteoarthritis.' The inference seems clear. Joints do not suffer if they are kept in regular use, but quickly deteriorate if they are allowed to remain idle. Osteoarthritis is therefore not caused by wear, as is so often thought, but by disuse.

This finding has been confirmed by research work carried out at Oxford University, which has revealed that the first part of a joint to become arthritic is not the part which is used most, but the part which is used least. Post-mortem studies show that the earliest signs of osteoarthritis in the hip occur in the cartilage lining the relatively little-used periphery of the joint rather than in the cartilage covering its weight-bearing centre. This is because regular exercise is necessary to ensure the adequate nutrition of the joint cartilage. When it is subjected to regular use the cartilage operates rather like a sponge, squeezing out its content of spent nutrient fluid whenever it is compressed, and then soaking up a fresh supply of nourishment from the rich network of blood vessels in the underlying bone whenever it is relieved of weight-bearing pressure. In this way the tissues are furnished with the foodstuffs necessary for tissue renewal and repair. This has been confirmed by injecting tracer dyes into the network of blood vessels lying under the cartilage. When the joints are used these dyes are quickly sucked up into the overlying cartilage, but no such diffusion of dye occurs if the joints are allowed to remain quiescent. Inactivity robs the cartilage of its essential supply of nourishment. As a result it rapidly atrophies. After seven weeks of total immobilization the cartilage shows an appreciable loss of both its resilience and its slipperiness. At a later stage, flakes of dead cartilage detach themselves from the joint surfaces and become a source of irritation to the capsule enclosing the joint. This gives rise to pain and protective muscle spasm which further increases the limitation of movement. Eventually the particles of dead cartilage adhere to the joint capsule where they become engulfed by layers of fibrous tissue. This makes them no longer a source of chronic irritation, but adds to the overall stiffness of the degenerating joint, which becomes increasingly prone to strain. Rising out of bed in the morning, or getting up from a chair is now a distinct problem. So too is bending down to put on a pair of socks or tights, climbing the stairs, or kneeling to weed the garden. Every added strain makes the muscles around the joint more tense, and increases the instinctive tendency to protect the damaged joint from further use. So the cycle of joint decay proceeds, as the diagram overleaf illustrates.

Some medical authorities believe that 95 per cent of the pain experienced during the early stages of osteoarthritis stems from protective muscle spasm and the growing stiffness of the capsule and periarticular tissues. This can be reversed. Animal experiments show that this early stiffness can be overcome, either by manipulative treatment or by self-administered exercise, although it may take as many as 200 days of active movement to overcome the pathological effects of thirty days of idleness. If at this stage we fail to take the necessary steps to restore the full mobility of our joints, the insidious process of joint

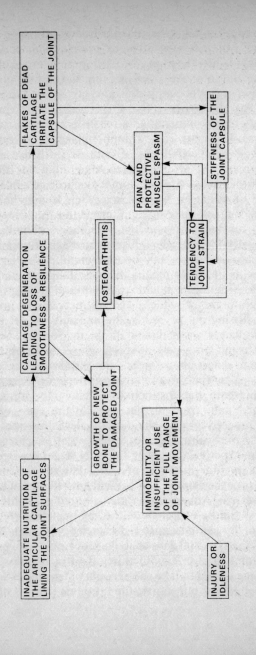

degeneration will progress until irreversible changes have occurred. But even then all hope is not lost. Many people with degenerative changes in their ankles, knees, backs and necks can derive considerable benefit from manipulative treatment, or from a well-planned course of mobilizing exercises.

Osteoarthritis is a chronic disease process largely because we take inadequate steps to check its progress. It overtakes people as they grow older, not because they have subjected their bodies to too much use, but because they have exercised their joints too little. People who practise daily yoga exercises ensure the proper nourishment of their joint tissues and are living proof that it is possible to remain remarkably supple and free from degenerative joint disease well into one's eighties and even nineties. The same benefits can be derived from carrying out the Reveille Ritual, described on pages 273–6.

Exercise, in addition to its prophylactic value in the prevention of muscular rheumatism, backache and osteoarthritis, also has an important part to play in the treatment of other rheumatic diseases which are less fully understood, such as rheumatoid arthritis and ankylosing spondylitis. At one time, patients stricken with rheumatoid arthritis were confined to bed and had their joints immobilized in plaster casts. Now it is realized that excessive recumbency only aggravates their problem. Even when the condition is at its height, and the joints exquisitely painful, an attempt should be made to put them gently through their full range of movements several times a day. This reduces the risk of adhesion formation, and limits the encroachment of connective tissue into the joint space. A similar policy is now adopted in the treatment of ankylosing spondylitis, a disease of unknown etiology, which often leads to progressive stiffening of the spine and the development of a 'poker' back. This was once managed by rest and anti-inflammatory drugs, which did little to check the progress of the disease or halt the creeping disability.

101

Now it is treated by active movement, with drugs used only to deaden the pain and make it easier to carry out the prescribed course of exercise. This has revolutionized the prognosis of the disease. Research carried out by the British army shows that soldiers suffering from ankylosing spondylitis have a 95 per cent chance of retaining the mobility of their spines and being able to continue with their jobs, providing they perform special spinal exercises every morning and night.

This confirms once more the importance of regular activity in the maintenance of joint health. Anyone who adopts the dynamogenic way of life outlined in this book will automatically provide himself with the finest panacea against rheumatic pain and joint disease. Those who are already victims of bad backs or stiff necks can accelerate their return to full health by adopting the following habits:

● *Keep active and purposefully occupied*. Rheumatic aches and pains are a built-in hazard of many jobs. It's difficult to avoid stiff necks and tension headaches if you're a desk-bound typist or office worker. The human head weighs about 4·5 kilos (10 lb). Holding it erect involves little muscular effort, providing the weight of the skull is carried directly over the spine. But tension is thrown on the supporting muscles of the neck the moment the head is allowed to droop forward like a water-logged boot dangling at the end of a fishing line. This is bound in time to produce neck pain – a problem which can be remedied by keeping the neck and shoulder muscles constantly on the move. Whenever desk workers pause for thought, they should develop the knack of closing their eyes, tipping their heads back and clasping their hands behind their necks. This will provide their necks with a few moments' respite from tension, and also give their colleagues an impressive display of studied concentration! In the same way copy typists should adopt the habit of alternating the side on which they hold their copy, so that their necks are not always twisted in the same direction. Sedentary workers should also make a point of seizing every opportunity during the day to quit their desks and indulge in other, more mobile, forms of activity. If a message has to be transmitted to a colleague in an office which is only a flight of stairs or a short corridor distance away, it is far better to deliver it personally than to try to make contact by inter-office phone. This positive action, apart from relieving the postural strain and tension in the trunk and limbs, is also often quicker and less frustrating than waiting for a switchboard connection followed by a response from an opposite number, who so abhors time wasting conversations with outsiders that he shows extreme reluctance in answering *any* call.

Many people try to avoid spinal aches and pains by equipping themselves with ergonomically designed desks and chairs, and adopting a 'correct' sitting position. These measures undoubtedly help to limit postural strains, but they cannot entirely eliminate them. It is a basic postural principle that no one position is ideal if it is maintained too long. Even if he is holding himself in an orthopaedically approved fashion, a guardsman will faint if he stands stock still for an excessive length of time. Sick patients develop bed sores, even in the most perfect hospital beds, unless their bodies are moved at regular intervals. In the same way desk workers will suffer painful backs and stiff necks even when they're sitting in expensive, scientifically designed executive desks and chairs, unless they change their posture from time to time.

The managers of a large chemical works in Germany succeeded in making an impressive improvement in the health of their typists by instigating a carefully planned programme of postural re-education. First, they equipped their offices with electric typewriters and specially designed typing chairs; then they limited their secretaries to six hours' typing a day. The rest of their time was to be spent in filing and other activities which took them away from their desks and enabled them to bend and stretch their spines. A masseuse was also employed to provide on-the-spot massage for tense, fibrositic muscles and to instruct the girls in loosening-up exercises. With this enlightened regime the efficiency of the girls increased and they suffered far fewer postural aches and pains.

Motorists should employ similar principles on long-distance drives. In recent years there has been a great improvement in the design of car seats which now give far more positive support for the back, but this has not eliminated the postural strain of driving. After two hours at the wheel of a car many motorists develop backache, stiff necks, tension headaches, neuritis in the arms, and sciatic pain in the legs, particularly in the right leg which is constantly held tense on the accelerator. This is because of the relatively fixed position of the body. With trunk pinioned in position by a restraint harness, hands locked to the steering wheel, head thrust aggressively forward peering intently at the road ahead and foot glued to the throttle, we have about as much room for manoeuvre as a trussed chicken. Sustaining this cramped position, particularly during tense road conditions, is a common cause of postural strain. This can be alleviated by making regular changes of posture. Even an occasional shift of weight from buttock to buttock can help to ease the strain of driving. Greater relief for the neck and shoulders can be obtained by making a ritual of dropping the hands from the steering wheel and turning the head from side to side whenever the car is stationary in a traffic jam or is brought to a halt at traffic lights. This helps to relieve the tension in the muscles of the arm and shoulders and ease the stiffness in the neck. Another valuable practice is to establish the habit of pulling into a lay-by or motorway service station after every ninety minutes of continuous driving to stretch the legs and exercise the trunk. A short while ago Opel, the German motor car manufacturers, hit upon the excellent idea of issuing motorists with a free chart of wayside exercises designed to counteract the harmful effects of long-distance driving. Most of these exercises required drivers to hold the car bonnet like a ballet dancer's barre, then swing their legs and flex their trunk from side to side. Performance of movements like these at regular intervals during a long journey can help to minimize strain and lessen fatigue.

Postural strains can also occur during the night. Few people realize just how dangerous it is to go to bed. Large numbers of back and neck injuries arise not during the day when we are lifting bags of cement or bumping grand pianos, but when we are lying innocently asleep and our spines are contorted in dangerous positions. This can largely be avoided by the use of suitable bedding. In the past, our ancestors slept quite comfortably on mats on the floor, on piles of fur rugs, or on straw-filled palliasses. Subsequent generations added upholstered divan bases, sprung mattresses and feather overlays in a misguided attempt to provide additional comfort, but this has only aggravated the risk of spinal strain. To have the maximum chance of a good night's rest, we need to sleep on a bed which is soft enough to cushion the body's bony parts, but firm enough to stop the spine sagging. Such a bed also facilitates the small shifts of posture that are necessary to stave off fatigue and prevent postural strain. Most people change their sleeping position anything from twenty to sixty times a night. If they didn't make these regular movements, areas of their skin would become sore from constant pressure, joints would be strained by being held on prolonged stretch and nerves made numb from constant compression. Beds need to be firm to make it possible to adopt a wide variety of poses and to ring the changes between them smoothly and easily. But there is no need to invest in expensive 'orthopaedic' beds which are sometimes twice as costly as ordinary beds and no more effective. The required degree of resilience can be obtained far more cheaply by placing a latex foam mattress on the floor or any other solid base.

● *Sit in chairs as little as possible.* A large percentage of backache stems from our habitual use of chairs. Many people today spend the majority of their lives in a cushioned throne, often of appalling design. They travel to work by bus, train or car; they are desk-bound for the majority of their working day and then spend their evenings slumped in front of a TV screen. A recent analysis of the daily routines of a group of forty adults shows that we spend an average of 69 per cent of our waking day sitting down, a figure which drops to 64 per cent at weekends. This prolonged inactivity predisposes us to obesity, coronary disease, backache, stiff necks, tension headaches, constipation, varicose veins and piles. The truth is that we are as ill-equipped for a sedentary existence as an elephant is for a life on the shifting ice floes of Antarctica. We are still not fully adapted to the standing posture which we adopted 800,000 years ago. What chance have we had to adjust to the sitting posture which we assumed no more than 5,000 years ago? This is only a blink in evolutionary time, and the only concession nature has made to our new mode of living is a slight thickening of the skin overlying the buttocks. Otherwise the structure of the human back and pelvis is just as it was when our ancestors were climbing trees and chasing game through the primeval forests. The resting poses they adopted then – kneeling, squatting, lying, and sitting cross-legged on the floor – put far less strain on the spine and provided far more postural change. Now when we sit we hold our bodies in virtually the same position for hours on end. Radiological studies have shown that when we sit with insufficient support for the small of the back, the lower two joints of the spine are tipped forwards as far as they will go. This means that two hours' sitting in a slumped position can produce as much postural strain as two hours' weeding in the garden.

The spinal discs also suffer in the sitting posture. When we are erect our abdominal muscles contract, which increases the intra-abdominal pressure and lessens the vertical loading on the spine. The moment we sit, we lose this natural uplift, with the result that the pressure on the spinal discs is twice as high in the sitting position as it is when standing. People with bad backs invariably find that they are most comfortable when they are on the move, and least happy when they are sitting down, particularly in soft easy chairs which provide as much support for their spines as a cream-filled meringue. Back sufferers would benefit if they dispensed with chairs altogether in the evening, and substituted instead a couch on which they could recline Roman fashion, or a few cushions sprinkled on the floor on which they could kneel, squat, lie prone, recline, crouch or sprawl. In this way, they would inevitably make regular shifts of posture throughout the evening.

Another way to escape the fatigue and postural strain of sitting is to use a rocking chair. In the opinion of Dr Barry Wyke, director of the Royal College of Surgeons' Neurological Unit, this is one of the finest ways of managing low back pains in elderly patients. 'My personal view,' he told a recent conference of osteopaths, 'is that the apparent increase in low back pain in this century compared with former times may be due to the disappearance of the rocking chair.' This was also the opinion of Dr Janet Travell who, during her time as physical medical consultant to the White House, advised President Kennedy to install a rocking chair in his personal office suite to ease his spinal pain. This is a measure she recommends to all back sufferers. 'The constantly changing position will relax your muscles and rest you,' she claims. Rhythmical swaying movements of the body always have a sedative effect, which is why mothers calm their children by rocking them in their arms and why the inmates of mental hospitals often console themselves by hugging their bodies and swaying slowly backwards and forwards. The same soothing effect can be obtained from the regular oscillations of a rocking chair, which has the advantage over tranquillizing drugs that it is cheap, easily obtained, has no side effects, is non-toxic and needs no prescription.

6

The Slim Gourmet

It is one of the cruel paradoxes of the twentieth century that while hordes of people in the Third World are dying from undernutrition, many of their more affluent neighbours are suffering from gross overnutrition. Obesity – the disease of conspicuous overconsumption and pampered indolence – has become a health hazard of epidemic proportions in all highly developed countries. It is believed that 35 million Americans and 5 million Britons are seriously overweight. Obesity, which has killed more people than the Black Death, is now a matter of governmental concern throughout the Western world. East German authorities estimate that fat people cost their country £60 million a year in unnecessary medical treatment, food wastage and industrial inefficiency. To combat this senseless drain of vital resources, Professor Hellmut Henel, director of one of the Republic's leading food research institutes, has recommended that the government should reduce the social benefits of everyone who is overweight. This would give encouragement to the ideal citizen whom the professor describes as being tall, slim, strong and mobile. But how many people today approach this ideal?

Most people put on weight as they grow older. Their thighs and buttocks grow pudgy, their waistline thickens and their jowls droop. This is so common that it was accepted in the past as an inevitable accompaniment of the ageing process. Early height/weight tables were usually based on measurements taken from a sample of nearly five million Americans, most of whom had become increasingly obese as they grew older through overeating and underexercising. A steady weight gain between the

109

ages of twenty and forty was naturally revealed when a computation was made of their average weights. This is a common finding, but one which is neither natural nor healthy. Unfortunately these norms are still accepted by some doctors when assessing a patient's 'ideal' weight. On the basis of these charts a 2-metre (6-ft) man is permitted to put on 6–8 kilos (15 lb) in weight between the ages of twenty-five and forty-five. But this extra poundage is due to the accumulation of fat and represents a health hazard far greater than smoking twenty-five cigarettes a day. There is no justification whatsoever for growing heavier with the passage of time. Body weight should reach a peak at about the age of twenty-five and, unless a prodigious amount of muscle-developing exercise is taken, should never afterwards rise above this level.

A person who is 10 per cent overweight is more than twice as likely to suffer symptoms of chronic ill health, such as fatigue, shortness of breath, indigestion, constipation and rheumatic aches and pains. Allow yourself to become fat and you're more likely to suffer a stroke, have 2½ times the risk of developing kidney disease, and 3½ times the risk of developing diabetes. It's impossible to be as fit as a fiddle when you're shaped like a double bass.

Knowing this, many people pursue crank ways of girth control. Thousands of housewives in France were beguiled recently into spending £365 on a set of magic saucepans, made of a 'health-giving mixture of chrome, steel and nickel', which the promoters claimed would help people keep 'fit and slim to the age of ninety-nine'. In fact the only virtue of these pans was that they were coated with a non-stick surface, which made it possible to fry foods without the addition of calorie-rich fats and oils. Others have submitted to having a staple driven through their ears, a weight control gimmick devised by Dr Lester Sacks, a family doctor from Los Angeles. He, and his two hundred specially trained staplepuncturists, have given a clip on the ear to scores of fatties in Britain and America, and claim that with its aid 75 per cent of patients have been enabled to shed 6 kilos (1 stone) or more in weight. Now, whenever they feel tempted to eat, instead of reaching for a jar of biscuits, they grasp their ear and twiddle furiously at the surgical staple. This is said to curb their hunger pangs, but no doubt other, less expensive, diversionary tactics would prove equally effective, such as going for a walk, taking up some knitting or making a cup of tea.

Then there are the wonder-working pills, injections and creams which are guaranteed to dispel your surplus inches like snow melting in the fierce heat of the sun. One remedy which enjoyed great popularity some years ago was a cream which, it was claimed, when applied to tubby tums, chubby chops and bulging butts was enough to make unwanted fat disappear. This miracle arose because the potion contained the active principle of marine plankton. Nobody needed telling that regular sea bathing is invigorating and slimming. What they didn't know, until the manufacturers of this cream bought extensive advertising space to enlighten them, was that this stimulus 'is due to the presence in sea water of marine plankton which acts on the metabolism.' The inference was that the simple act of rubbing plankton extract on to the skin would raise the level of metabolism and so burn up the body's stores of fat. The theory must have convinced many people, who seemed as willing to part with their excess cash as they were eager to lose their surplus weight. But the sales spiel overlooked two salient facts. As far as is known plankton contains no ingredients capable of raising the rate of human metabolism, and even if it did they would not be able to penetrate the barrier provided by the skin. Anyone wanting to enjoy a course of marine slimming would be better employed skinny dipping in the briny than dipping their skin in cream. If you follow any of these slimming gimmicks the only thing that will become lighter is your bank balance.

For the desperately overweight there are a variety of

surgical operations. Some have had their jaws wired together for weeks on end, so that they have had to survive on a liquid diet, and have been unable to indulge their craving for popcorn, pastries and pasta. Others have submitted to a jejunal by-pass operation, which effectively removes from use 18 to 20 feet of the intestinal tract. This device undoubtedly reduces the amount of nourishment absorbed by the gut, but seems an unnecessarily drastic measure of calorie control, particularly as the operation carries a 4 per cent mortality rate.

More popular still are the endless variety of calorie controlled diets, varying from the one-food-each-day-a-week diet to the if-it-tastes-good-spit-it-out diet and the steak-three-times-a-day-straight-way-to-bankruptcy diet. These diets have only one thing in common – they don't work. Experience shows that only twelve out of every hundred overweight people going on a low-calorie diet can expect to lose significant amounts of weight after a year's stringent dieting, and of these favoured dozen only two will retain their weight loss by the end of the following year. The remainder will be victims of the yo-yo syndrome, their weight swinging wildly up and down as they vainly pursue a succession of Scarsdale diets, Hollywood diets, fruit-juice-only diets, and *cuisine minceur*. Some regimes tell them to eat as much fruit as they like, others, like Dr Pennington's, warn them that they will put on weight if they so much as look at half an apple. This great dietary disaster, instead of encouraging people to look for other ways of getting slim, merely stimulates them to look for alternative diets which with incredible optimism they always believe will be more effective than the ones they've tried before. But disappointment is bound to follow. As the famous nutritionalist Gayelord Hauser writes, 'In more than thirty years' helping oversized people return to normal, I have never known a single case of overweight to be brought under *permanent* control *by a low-calorie* diet alone.'

Trying to keep slim on a calorie-reduced diet is rather

like sailing through life in a leaky barge – there's never an end to the perpetual chore of baling out. Eating is a joyful, convivial act, whereas dieting is anti-social and unpleasant. The Greek gods lived on ambrosia, the Jews look forward to a land flowing with milk and honey, but the only temptations offered to modern slimmers are the synthetic delights of starch reduced rolls, diuretic pills, artificial sweeteners, and methylcellulose chips to swell the stomach and produce a false sensation of satiety. What a grim future to envisage! Eating stripped of all its epicurean pleasure.

But it's not necessary to follow a life of constant asceticism to stay healthy and slim. People who adopt the dynamogenic life style can dine on duck pâté, lobster thermidor, poached salmon, crêpes Suzette, and strawberry mousse, washed down with the finest clarets and burgundies and still remain slim, lithe and energetic. Why be eternally counting calories when you can leave your internal computer to maintain the body's metabolic balance sheet? Why chew ice cubes to stave off your hunger pangs when you can slake your appetite with a mouth-watering casserole? Eating is for pleasure as well as nutrition, just as sex is for fun as well as procreation. So why deny yourself the second greatest pleasure in life, when there's another, simpler way of keeping in trim – particularly when it's so obvious that stringent dieting does not work as a long-term method of weight control?

Crash diets are doomed to failure because they're invariably unbalanced, dull, anti-social and nutritionally unsound. In an attempt to lose weight many people give up eating bread and potatoes, but these are both vital ingredients in our diet. About a quarter of our total protein intake comes from bread, and during the winter potatoes may supply as much as a third of our total intake of Vitamin C. Malnutrition can arise if these essential foodstuffs are shunned and no adequate replacements found. Others try to lose weight and reduce their overall intake of cholesterol by cutting down their intake of dairy

113

foods. But this too can prove a nutritional mistake, for dairy products are a valuable source of protein and currently provide a quarter of our total intake of calcium. People who go on low-calorie diets can also suffer a loss of drive. This lowered vitality slows them down and reduces their consumption of energy – a pointless economy for dieters anxious to burn up their surplus stores of fat. Dieting is self-defeating if it produces fatigue and a resultant decline in activity. Tests show that people who go on a fast reduce their basal metabolic rate by as much as 20 per cent. This means that they can maintain their body weight on a vastly decreased intake of calories.

Strict dieting can also have a devastating effect on the body's normal mechanism for appetite regulation and control. Doctors who have no weight problems often fail to realize how hungry their dieting patients become. Empty stomachs become the site of tantalizing hunger pangs, so much so that it becomes an agonizing ordeal to pass a baker's shop and feast the eyes, but nothing else, on shelves laden with iced buns and chocolate éclairs. Slimmers may give up their breakfasts, and take a meagre lunch of a hard-boiled egg (one only because of its high cholesterol content), a few slices of tomato (no more because the oxalic acid they contain may favour the formation of kidney stones) and a few leaves of lettuce (unadorned by mayonnaise dressing which is far too fattening). But as their blood sugar level falls they feel a craving to eat something sweet. To satisfy this longing they take an illicit sweetened coffee, a few biscuits, and one or two sweets. This gives their blood sugar level an immediate boost, but also stimulates the pancreas to secrete more insulin, which takes some of the excess sugar out of circulation and keeps the blood sugar level within reasonable limits. Unfortunately, this response is sometimes overdone, particularly when high calorie snacks are taken on an empty stomach. As a result, too much sugar is taken out of the bloodstream and converted into fat. This adds to the body's stores of fat and causes the blood sugar level to plummet rapidly, leading to more fatigue and further craving for sugary tit-bits and highly concentrated sweetened foods. In this way even the most dedicated slimmers, while desperately trying to reduce their calorie consumption, are faced with the constant urge to satisfy their hunger and overcome their tiredness by eating calorie-rich, between-meal snacks. This is one reason why people find it so difficult to adhere to low-calorie diets.

Some years ago Dr Albert J. Stukard, Chairman of the Department of Psychiatry at the University of Pennsylvania, analysed the results of eight carefully conducted weight-reducing programmes and concluded, 'Results of treatment for obesity are remarkably similar and remarkably poor.' He fared little better when he supervized his own slimming programme at the Nutrition Clinic of New York Hospital. At the end of a year's stringent dieting he found that only 6 per cent of his patients had achieved a satisfactory weight loss, and by the end of the second year he could claim no more than a 2 per cent success rate.

It is not surprising that the resolve of many dieters fails when they are faced with the promptings of a healthy but unsatisfied appetite. If there is a conflict between the physiological craving to eat and an intellectual desire to refrain from eating, the biological urge will invariably win. In fact, considering the artificial, indolent lives we lead, the remarkable thing is not that some people become grossly fat, but that the majority of people put on so little weight throughout their lives. Think of the wide variation in our calorie intake and output. We may be poor and unable to find the money to pay for a decent meal, or we may be a wealthy tycoon forced to eat an endless succession of rich meals at lavish, expense account restaurants. We may be a six-foot labourer living by the sweat of our brow, or a dainty seven-stone dowager waited on by a retinue of servants. We may be a growing child, a pregnant mother, a wheelchair cripple

115

or an international athlete. Whatever our metabolic status, our body performs a remarkably efficient job in balancing our food intake according to our energy needs. Between the ages of twenty-five and sixty-five the normal woman eats about 20 tons of food but puts on an average of only 24 lb in weight. This represents an error of only 3½ ounces of food a year in excess of requirements, or considerably less than half a chip a day too much. This denotes a remarkably accurate balancing of the metabolic ledger, and an incredibly close matching of energy demand and supply. Just suppose that an average woman developed a craving for chocolate layer cake and from the age of twenty-five onwards couldn't resist taking a daily two-inch slice of this tempting delicacy over and above her true calorie requirements. Taking a surplus 450 calories a day she would theoretically put on 18 kilos (40 lbs) a year and reach a gargantuan weight of over a tonne by the time she reached the age of sixty-five, were it not for the fact that her body has a highly efficient weight-controlling mechanism, which overrides her compulsive desire to eat and keeps her shape within manageable proportions.

For several decades scientists searched for the location of this appetite-regulating centre. They knew it must exist even though it did not seem to act as accurately as the mechanisms which control other essential bodily functions such as blood pressure, the beating of the heart, the acidity of the blood, the rate of respiration or the level of blood sugar. Eventually they located it in part of the mid brain known as the hypothalamus, and nicknamed it the 'appestat'. Experiments showed that if this vital centre was destroyed in laboratory rats, the animals overate and became obese. But if the centre remained intact, the animals could be given unlimited food to eat and would always eat just sufficient to balance their metabolic needs without becoming fat. There was no need for them to count their calories, stop eating potatoes, ride static bicycles, eat starch-reduced bread or wear special slimming garments. Providing their appestat was functioning, the rats could eat whatever they fancied without becoming obese. This automatic weight-controlling mechanism is present in rats, cats, dogs, monkeys and man, and is as essential for the preservation of life as the homeostatic devices which Nature provides to regulate the heart rate and blood pressure. After all what's the point of being protected from heart failure and strokes only to die from being overweight? If we observe its dictates, the body contains all that is necessary to preserve our life, health and vigour, without the need for calorie control and constant dietary supervision.

To tackle obesity successfully, it's necessary to work *with* Nature, rather than *against* her. This means making full and proper use of the appestat, rather than employing futile attempts to curb the body's perfectly natural desire to eat delicious foods. Get your appestat working properly, and you can forget about dieting for the rest of your life.

Many researchers have tried to discover what it is that makes us feel replete. They believe that they will be able to control obesity if they can only discover the signals that make the appestat aware when our energy requirements have been met. Do our satiety centres respond to the level of glucose in the blood, or are they responsive to other chemical stimuli, such as the level of circulating gastric hormones or essential fatty acids? Answer this question, the pharmaceutical research workers say, and it may be possible to develop a drug which tricks the hypothalamus into prematurely thinking that it's had enough. But while this advance may prove highly profitable to the drug industry, it will not eradicate the problem of obesity. It will merely introduce a new form of treatment, substituting continuous drug therapy for lifelong dietary control. The most important facts about the appestat have already been revealed. Experiments show that the appestat works effectively, accurately matching calorie input and output, only when energy output exceeds a certain minimum level. Just as the automatic exposure meter on a camera will only operate when there is a certain minimum level of light, so the appetite-regulating centres in the brain can only function properly when activity exceeds a certain optimum level. This was discovered at Edinburgh University when dogs were given varying degrees of exercise and unlimited amounts of food. Repeated tests showed that providing the dogs were sufficiently energetic, they ate only sufficient to keep their weight steady. But if their activity was artificially curbed, their appetite-regulatory mechanism failed to operate effectively, with the result that they overate and became obese. The same breakdown is likely to occur in humans. As the Edinburgh research workers surmized, 'The daily physical activity of many thousands of light workers may be below the threshold needed for appetite to function normally. For this reason they may overeat and become obese.'

The same conclusion was reached by Dr Jean Mayer, the eminent American nutritionalist, who carried out a similar series of experiments on laboratory rats at the Department of Nutrition of the Harvard University School of Public Health. He gave all the rats an unlimited supply of food, but kept some in a state of enforced idleness, while giving others varying amounts of exercise from one to eight hours a day. Analysis revealed that less than one hour's exercise a day is insufficient to activate a rat's appetite-regulating mechanism. Animals who took less exercise than this consumed too much food and became increasingly fat, while those who got more than an hour's activity a day automatically matched their calorie input and output, and so mainained a steady weight. Studies in India suggest that exactly the same considerations apply to humans. Surveys conducted by the Harvard research team showed that Indians who perform active manual jobs have little difficulty remaining slim, whereas their more sedentary compatriots tend to put on weight and cannot rely on the satiety cenres in their brains to regulate their appetites. As Dr Mayer concluded, 'In the US most of us are down in the sedentary range, where the regulators [in the brain] don't work very well for most people.'

If we want to escape the need for constant dieting we must lead more active lives. This is the only natural way of weight control. People put on weight as they grow older not because they increase their consumption of food, but because they decrease their level of activity. This is the reason for the ubiquitous middle-aged spread.

Surveys show that many fat adults actually eat less than their slim neighbours. They grow obese only because they lead excessively sedentary lives. At forty we don't run up the stairs quite as fast as we did in our teens. Instead of taking an active part in sport we're content to sit back and watch it on TV. When we go to a dinner/dance we devote more time to the dinner and far less to the dance. Our love life is less frequent and somewhat more sedate, our hobbies more passive, our excitement less acute. By middle age we are probably burning up 15 to 20 per cent fewer calories than we did when we were twenty, but only rarely do we make the necessary adjustment in our calorie intake. So we become fat. The average sedentary individual puts on about a pound of surplus weight a year once he passes the age of twenty-five. This gradual growth in girth is unsightly, unhealthy and uncomfortable, and could be prevented by taking no more than an extra three minutes' walking a day. The classic middle-age spread is caused not by gluttony but by sloth.

A few years ago the Canadian Federal Government was shocked by a report which revealed the poor state of the nation's health. The average thirty-year-old Canadian male, it was found, was no fitter than the average sixty-year-old Swede. Over half the adult Canadian population was overweight. This was attributable to the increasing passivity of Canadian life. Researchers discovered that

119

there was little variation in the calorie intake of fat Canadians and those who maintained a healthy weight. The main difference lay in their level of activity. So the Government instigated a nationwide fitness campaign, called Sport Participation Canada, aimed at getting the nation back on its feet. This was so successful that on one freezing winter's night 60,000 inhabitants of Saskatoon, in Saskatchewan – a remarkable 51 per cent of the population – responded to the call to drop whatever they were doing and walk around the block. Providing the Saskatoons continue to take their daily walk around the block they've got the problem of obesity licked.

For years health authorities throughout the Western world have been barking up the wrong tree. They've been encouraging their overweight citizens to stop eating, when they should have been urging them to start exercising instead. In 1958 the Food and Nutrition Board of the American National Academy of Sciences recommended that, to remain healthy and slim, the average American male should consume 3200 calories a day and the average female 2300. A few years later the Board recognized that this allowance was too generous. Technological changes had made the life of the average American far less energetic. Labour-saving gadgets were replacing horsepower for muscle power on the domestic front, while outside the home the development of motorized transport – drive-in cinemas, drive-in banks, and even drive-in mortuaries – were conspiring to make legs obsolete. Like destiny, the motor car was shaping Uncle Sam's ends, both metaphorically and literally. Faced with this rapid decline in physical activity, what did the Board recommend? Logically it should have launched a sports participation programme, and issued a call for a return to a more vigorous way of life. Instead it made an ineffectual call to Americans to tighten their belts and endeavour to reduce their food intake still further to 2300 calories a day in the case of the average-sized male, and 2100 calories a day in the case of Ms

Average America. This improved the well-being of the thousands of firms making low calorie foods, slimming aids and sugar substitutes, but did little to enhance the nation's health.

Calorie-restricted diets may produce a temporary loss of weight, but they cannot achieve a positive state of health. You won't tighten up flabby muscles by dieting, nor can you improve the function of your heart and lungs by stopping eating potatoes and bread. But if you adopt a dynamogenic lifestyle you'll find you not only lose weight painlessly and permanently, but in addition you gain energy, improve your circulation, feel happier, and enjoy a livelier sex life. But don't expect to find this message emblazoned on roadside hoardings and throughout the pages of the glossy magazines. There are millions of pounds to be made by encouraging people to wage a constant dietary battle against overweight, and nothing to be derived from showing them how to stay permanently slim and healthy by adopting a more vital way of life. Powerful vested interests want you to carry on the soulless task of counting calories. You are the only beneficiary, plus your family and friends, when you practice the art of dynamogenic living.

This is a habit which should be established early in life. One of the most important lessons we can teach our children is to lead exciting, active and productive lives. Lazy parents tend to breed idle children. Surveys show that when both parents are fat, three-quarters of their offspring are similarly overweight – a risk which is more than eight times greater than that for children of slim parents. This is largely due to a difference in exercise levels – a pattern acquired during the youngster's formative years.

Dr Jean Mayer and his co-workers at Harvard University took a group of twenty-eight overweight schoolgirls and compared their diet and schedule of activities with a similar number of girls who were of normal weight, but were otherwise matched as closely as possible as regards age, height and position in class. They found that the fat girls actually ate a little less than their classmates, and put on weight simply because they led far less active lives. They spent four times as many hours a day watching television, and took only a third as much exercise – swimming, walking, dancing and competitive sports – as the girls of normal weight. In another study Dr Mayer took cine pictures of nearly two hundred girls of all shapes and sizes playing volleyball, tennis and swimming. Careful analysis of these films showed that when fat girls take part in sport, they do so in a way which is far less vigorous than girls of normal weight. As a result they burn up fewer calories.

This is one of the great problems of obesity. Once the layers of fat have been deposited, they're extremely difficult to shift. Fat people find it difficult to run up and down stairs, so they take the lift or make their ascent at a more leisurely pace. Since they get out of breath on the slightest exertion, they give up hurrying after buses, chasing dogs, riding bikes, playing tennis and dancing anything more lively than a slow tempo waltz. They complain that their feet are killing them, but in fact they're killing their overloaded feet, which become so uncomfortable that they reduce their standing and walking to a minimum. Doctors give fat children notes to excuse them from taking part in school sports and physical training activities. As a result, their lives become more and more sedentary. When they take a seaside vacation fatties are too embarrassed to expose their mountainous flesh to public view, so they sit muffled up in a deckchair, reading a book, chewing sweets and eating ice-creams, while others play ball games on the beach and frolic in the sea. So they grow steadily fatter. This makes it easier for them to conserve the thermal energy of the body, since fat provides three times as much insulation against heat loss as muscle. As a result they can keep warm on cold days with relatively little expenditure of energy. Tests show that exposure to cold may increase the metabolism of lean subjects by 11 to 16 per cent, but may cause an increase of only 2½ per cent in the fuel consumption of people swathed in a duffle coat of fat.

Everything conspires to keep fat people fat. The Federation of Fatties is an easy club to join, but a difficult one to quit. Many people try to relinquish their right to membership by stringent dieting, but most fail. Some lose no weight on a diet so sparse that it wouldn't satisfy an anorexic sparrow. Even after weeks of vigorous self-denial they fail to lose a single ounce of flab. Their doctors assume they've been cheating on their diet. And when they plaintively announce that they've been eating like a bird, their friends immediately assume that the bird they're referring to is a vulture. But the fact remains that some people can retain their excess weight on the most meagre diets. Tests show that prolonged dieting can lead to a reduction in the body's need for food, so that standard 'slimming' diets cease to be effective. When doctors measured the food intake of a group of 905 teenagers attending schools in Berkeley, California, they discovered that the average calorie consumption of boys of normal weight was 3,000 calories a day, and for girls 2,060 calories a day. The average calorie intake of overweight youngsters in the group, far from exceeding this figure, was actually about 25 per cent less (2,360 calories a day for the fat boys and 1,530 a day for the fat girls). And even though these hapless Billy and Bessie Bunters continued to eat less than their slim classmates, they went on getting fatter during the course of the three-year study.

Energy utilization studies performed at Oxford University reveal that some unfortunate people have an abnormally low rate of metabolism and burn up only half as much energy as others when lying, sitting and standing. This means that they can eat half as many calories as people of normal weight and still remain obese.

123

This was confirmed by a fascinating trial carried out in 1975 by research workers attached to Queen Elizabeth College, London. Volunteers for this experiment were recruited from 8,000 women attending slimming clubs throughout the country. From this group twenty-nine guinea-pigs were selected, who had all adhered to a strict reducing diet for more than six months, but had been unable to shed weight, apart from a modest loss in the first few weeks. These recalcitrant reducers were taken to Ragdale Hall, an isolated country house in Leicestershire, and placed on a strict reducing diet which supplied them with an average of 1,350 calories a day. When they arrived their baggage was searched to see that they weren't smuggling in supplies of biscuits, cakes and sweets, and during the course of their stay they were kept under close observation to make sure that they weren't raiding the larder, or in any other way obtaining illicit supplies of food. At the end of three weeks' dieting under the strictest possible medical surveillance, their weights were taken and it was discovered that nine of the women had failed to lose weight, while three had actually added to their bulk! Subsequent tests showed that the women who hadn't lost weight all possessed abnormally low metabolic rates. To ask such people to lose weight by making further reductions in their intake of food is to sentence them to a life of constant abnegation. This approach also runs the risk of placing them on diets which are nutritionally deficient in other respects. The only sensible solution to their problem is to help them increase their rate of metabolism. This can be done with drugs, such as thyroxine which increases the rate of general bodily metabolism, or flenfluramine which increases the rate of peripheral metabolism. But slimming pills often produce harmful side effects, rarely secure more than a temporary loss of weight, and are no long-term solution to the problem of obesity. The only safe and acceptable way for these people to achieve permanent mastery of their weight problem is to increase the vitality of their lives. This will keep them both slim and healthy.

Some people may be unfortunate in inheriting a low metabolic rate, which means they have a constant tendency to put on weight. But this doesn't mean they've got to *remain* fat. Even if your mother was fat, your father fat, your grandparents gross, and every one of your ancestors back to Methuselah enormous, it still doesn't mean that you have to be overweight. Follow the dynamogenic programme outlined in this book and you can maintain a sylph-like figure without the need for constant dieting.

Sceptics will try to deter you by pointing out the prodigious amounts of exercise that have to be taken to lose 0.5 kilos (1 lb) in weight. And it's perfectly true that you've got to walk 54 km (34 miles) or swim non-stop for eight hours, to lose 0.5 kilos of fat. These may seem impossible tasks. But nobody suggests that all this activity has got to be taken in a single day. Step up your level of exercise throughout the entire year and you'll hardly notice the effort of losing weight. Take an extra half hour's stroll a day and you'll burn up 5 kilos (12 lb) of fat by the end of a year, and feel immeasurably fitter as a result. Have a half-hour's swim three times a week and you'll shed another 6 kilos (14 lb) a year, and in the process gain a figure which you'll be more proud to display in a bathing costume. And don't believe the pessimists who say that all this healthy exercise will merely increase your appetite, and so keep you as plump as ever. It's undoubtedly true that if you spend the morning at the golf course, and end up taking a couple of pints of beer and a large cheese sandwich at the nineteenth hole, you'll practically compensate for the energy expended during your three-hour round of golf, but you'd probably have had the ploughman's lunch in any case, even if you'd only spent the morning idly driving round the countryside in your car. Besides, experience shows that most people who take up vigorous outdoor exercise do not develop such massive appetites that they replace in the dining room what they've lost on the sports field.

Dr Kenneth Cooper, originator of the United States Air Force Aerobics training programme, finds that the appetite of many people actually drops when they take up vigorous sport. As he says, 'Such exercise shunts the blood away from your stomach. As a result you don't have the desire for food. Even after you've recovered from the exercise, your appetite rarely increases above normal. The net result is that you tend to eat less without feeling hungry.' This effect is less noticeable following mild exercise. After a long walk in the brisk country air it's normal to experience a quickening of the appetite, but the well-earned meal that follows is rarely enough to replace the extra calories consumed. According to Dr Grant Gwinup, Director of the Metabolic Research Laboratory at the University of California, the increase in appetite after taking moderate exercise rarely replaces more than about 60 per cent of the additional energy consumed. This means that after an hour and a half's game of tennis it's possible to tuck into a meal which includes such additional delicacies as a bowl of steaming mulligatawny soup, a crisp potato baked in its jacket and topped with a knob of butter, a glass of lager and a generous slice of cheese cake – and still lose weight! How much better than sitting in front of the television set and growing stiff, stout and stale on an insipid diet of clear celery soup, low-fat cheese, lettuce leaves and a cup or two of saccharine-sweetened black coffee.

And there's another benefit of exercise that's often overlooked when the rival merits of various forms of weight control are discussed. Physical activity greatly increases the rate at which we burn up fuel, and this effect does not stop the moment we cease exercising as so many people think, but continues for some while after-wards, albeit at a gradually diminishing rate. This means that if you go for a jog in the evening, and come home to a shower, a brisk rub-down and a quiet read by the fireside, you'll still be losing weight even while you're cosily relaxed in your easy chair! Take sufficient spells of activity during the day and your metabolic rate will remain permanently raised. In this way you can live well, feel well and stay well, without the need to apply a constant artificial curb on your appetite.

This is not an airy promise, but a solid fact backed by numerous experiments. Moderate exercise, such as walking, housework and carpentry, doubles the rate of bodily metabolism, whilst strenuous exercise such as sawing wood and playing tennis can produce a ten-fold increase or more in the resting rate of metabolism. As a result, sportsmen can eat prodigious amounts of food without the slightest risk of getting fat. In preparation for the 1978 Inter-varsity boat race, each member of the Cambridge University crew ate over 6,500 calories a day but did not put on an ounce of surplus weight. During the height of their training their typical breakfast menu provided more calories than a slimmer receives in a day, and included generous helpings of orange juice, porridge, a heaped plateful of bacon, eggs and sausages, toast, marmalade and unlimited quantities of milk. At the same time the Oxford crew dined on Barbados sugared ham baked in cider and orange juice, Persian chicken stuffed with apricots, or moussaka rich with potatoes, cheese and lashings of cream. In between times they feasted on everything that is taboo to the serious dieter – meringues, biscuits, toffee bars, cheese cake, flapjacks, bread and chocolate layer cake. But they didn't put on so much as a globule of fat, because they rowed off every delicious calorie they ate.

Long-distance swimmers can also eat large quantities of food without becoming fat. People who claim that it's impossible to lose weight by exercising obviously haven't tried swimming the English Channel. When Antonio Albertondo, the long-distance Argentinian swimmer, swam both ways across the English Channel in a non-stop time of forty-three hours, his physiological responses were monitored by a team of doctors from the National Institute of Medical Research, London. They found that during his marathon swim he burnt up 32,000 calories. While in the water he kept up his strength by taking occasional snacks of chicken broth, fruit and sandwiches. Despite this he lost 6 kilos (14 lb) in weight during the double crossing, most of which came from his stores of body fat.

Maybe you can't row, have an antipathy for water, and are not too enthusiastic about taking forty-three hours of non-stop strenuous exercise. If so, take heart. There are many far less arduous ways of working off your excess weight. A daily stint of walking is one such technique. Dr Gwinup proved this when he gave a group of eleven overweight women a programme of progressive walking exercise. During the course of the experiment they were free to eat what they liked and as much as they liked without restriction of any kind. All they were asked to do was to go for a daily walk of gradually increasing length. On this regime every woman lost a reasonable amount of weight, and maintained the loss for a year or more. Not surprisingly the results achieved were closely linked with the amount of exercise taken. The average loss was 9 kilos (22 lb), but the more conscientious women lost as much as 17 kilos (38 lb), while others who spent less time on their daily constitutional lost only 4 kilos (10 lb). One interesting finding of the study is that it appears to be necessary to walk at least half an hour a day to register an appreciable weight loss.

Many of Dr Gwinup's patients admitted that they would rather stay at home than go for their daily stride round the block. But all agreed that they were pleased with their weight loss, and delighted with the sense of relaxation and enhanced well-being they derived from their regular exercise. This was in direct contrast to the ennervation they had experienced in the past from dieting, which had tended to leave them feeling tired, weak and irritable, even if they did lose weight.

If you urgently need to lose weight, and are tired of struggling with an endless succession of unsuccessful slimming diets, start to follow the dynamogenic way of life. This will automatically restore you to a healthy weight by changing your entire metabolic balance, as the diagram overleaf shows. By following the first step of the dynamogenic programme outlined in the last chapter of this book you will increase the number of calories you burn up in healthy exercise during your leisure hours; by pursuing the programme's second step you will consume more energy maintaining your body temperature, and by following the fourth step you will increase the amount of nervous energy you expend. This, as well as revitalizing your life, will also help you to re-establish a healthy calorie balance and overcome your constant tendency to put on weight.

Also try to observe the following habits:

● *Keep active and purposefully occupied.* Dieting fails partly because of its negative approach. A strong will is invariably more effective than a strong won't. As a result it's generally easier to take something up than to give something up. So instead of cutting down calorie input, try stepping up calorie output. Try to inject more activity into every hour of your waking day. Standing, for instance, burns up five more calories an hour than sitting. So if you're an office worker, and spend three quarters of an hour a day on the telephone, you can burn up about a pound of unwanted fat a year simply by refusing to be chairbound when you take your calls. By pacing gently round your desk you'll also help to ease some of the postural strain of prolonged sitting. Again, since walking up and down stairs uses up five times as much energy as standing still, you can burn up an extra three hundred calories a week by shunning lifts and escalators and getting an extra ten minutes

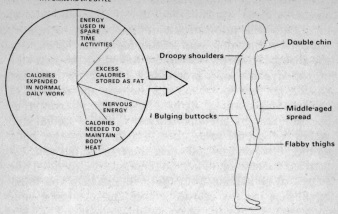

HYPOKINETIC LIFE STYLE

ENERGY USED IN SPARE TIME ACTIVITIES

EXCESS CALORIES STORED AS FAT

CALORIES EXPENDED IN NORMAL DAILY WORK

NERVOUS ENERGY

CALORIES NEEDED TO MAINTAIN BODY HEAT

Droopy shoulders

Double chin

Bulging buttocks

Middle-aged spread

Flabby thighs

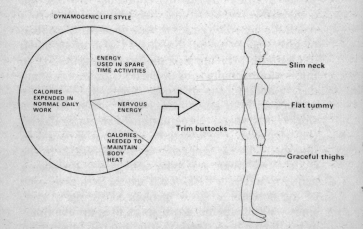

DYNAMOGENIC LIFE STYLE

ENERGY USED IN SPARE TIME ACTIVITIES

CALORIES EXPENDED IN NORMAL DAILY WORK

NERVOUS ENERGY

CALORIES NEEDED TO MAINTAIN BODY HEAT

Slim neck

Flat tummy

Trim buttocks

Graceful thighs

walking a day. This will also help to trim the muscles of your legs.

Similarly, if you knit, sew or whittle away at a piece of wood while watching TV you can burn up an extra twenty calories an hour, which could make you over a kilogram lighter by the end of the year. Better still, sit yourself in a rocking chair and spend the evening swaying gently backwards and forwards in your chair. If you spend three hours a night watching TV you will burn up over 14,000 more calories a year if you keep your body moving in a rocking chair, than if you sit passively in a conventional fireside chair. This is equivalent to a loss of over four pounds of surplus fat a year. Rocking will also improve the circulation and help to ease the aches and pains in your shoulders, back and neck.

If you commute to work by bus or tube try to get off one stop before your office and cover the rest of the trip on foot. Do the same when you're travelling to the shops. If you use a car on these occasions, park it a few blocks away from your final destination and walk the remainder of the journey. This may give you the opportunity to burn up another eighty calories a day, which translates into a loss of a further eight pounds a year. In this way your weight will slowly, but inexorably, decline.

Try particularly to get some gentle movement soon after eating a meal. It's usually said that it's unwise to exercise too soon after eating a hearty meal. But far sounder advice is to avoid eating meals which are so heavy that you can't get up from the table immediately afterwards and climb a flight of stairs or run for a bus. Heavy meals will make you feel disinclined to exercise. They'll also draw blood to the actively working digestive organs and leave that much less to supply the muscles, brain and heart. This can predispose to cramp, lethargy and coronary disease. Far better to take lighter, more easily digested meals, which place no strain on the body's circulatory system, and leave you feeling fresh enough to take an after-dinner dance instead of a post-prandial snooze. This will also increase the rate at which you burn up fuel. Eating normally acts as a stimulus to metabolism, but this effect is doubled if exercise is taken directly after a meal. Professor Yudkin and his colleagues at the Department of Nutrition and Dietetics, London University, confirmed this by studying the responses of a group of eleven young adults who were overfed for periods varying from one to two months. Tests revealed that after taking a 1,000-calorie meal the youngsters' metabolic rate showed an average increase of 28 per cent when they remained idle in a chair, but rose by 56 per cent when they took a half-hour's exercise. This increased metabolic activity helped to limit their gain in weight.

● *Eat more frequently, whenever you feel hungry.* Dietary studies show that people who are slim tend to spread their calorie intake more evenly during the day than fat people, who are prone to indulge their love of food by having one or two large binges a day rather than a series of smaller snacks. This orgiastic pattern of eating may contribute to their weight gain for two main reasons. In the first place, after a heavy meal the level of fat and glucose in the bloodstream soars. This stimulates the pancreas to secrete more insulin to take some of the surplus calories out of the circulation and place them in the body's fuel reserves of fat. In addition, since the mere fact of eating elevates the body's metabolic rate by 20 to 30 per cent, the person who takes more regular meals experiences several food-induced peaks of metabolism during the day instead of only one or two. This can burn up an additional two hundred calories a day.

132

Experience shows that if you want to remain slim it's better to be a nibbler than a gobbler. Dr Clarence Cohn of the Michael Reese Hospital, Chicago demonstrated this when he gave two groups of 750 white rats identical quantities of food, and allowed one group to nibble their quota of food whenever they wanted throughout the day, while the other was made to consume their rations in two set meals. Although both groups of rats ate exactly the same number of calories, it was found that after forty-one days the enforced gobblers had accumulated almost twice as much fat as the nibblers. This is an important metabolic discovery for tubby humans as well as rotund rats. If you find it desperately difficult to lose weight on a calorie controlled diet, try raising your rate of metabolism by spreading your intake of calories over five or six meals a day, instead of the traditional two or three. Professor Dorothy Pringle, of the Department of Nutritional Science at the University of Wisconsin-Madison, tested this technique by taking six women students who were at least 23 per cent overweight and placing them on a 1,300-calorie diet spread out over six meals a day. On this regime all the girls lost weight at the rate of 1–2 kilos (2–5 lb) a week without feeling particularly hungry. As an added bonus they also reported that they had 'more energy' than before they started dieting.

Trials in Czechoslovakia have also shown that people who consume five or six meals a day have a significantly lower blood cholesterol level than those who limit their intake of food to three or fewer meals a day. This reduction in blood fats probably lowers their risk of cardiovascular disease, which is a valuable reward for so minor a change in dietary habit. To go on the 'Nibbler's Diet' all that's necessary is to have a modest breakfast and lunch and a lighter than usual dinner, and then take

133

additional snacks in the mid-morning and mid-afternoon which can consist of an apple and cheese, a wholemeal biscuit and a small glass of milk or a handful of nuts and raisins. On this regimen, providing you don't increase your overall intake of calories, you'll find it easier to lose weight, you'll get less hungry, and you'll enjoy a higher level of vitality.

● *Be enthusiastic about all you do.* Metabolism can be increased not only by eating more frequent meals, but also by enjoying a life which is emotionally more vigorous and lively. Fat people are often depicted as being cheerful, jolly extroverts, but personality studies show that more often than not they are withdrawn, prone to depression, and burdened with guilt about their unsightly appearance and uncontrolled pattern of eating. When a team of psychiatrists and psychologists from the New England Medical Centre, Boston, compared the personality of 135 fat women and 80 women of normal weight, they found that the obese women were noticeably more tense, more withdrawn, less inclined to make friends, more prone to daydreaming, and more given to witholding their feelings for others, either of anger or affection. If these inhibited individuals can be encouraged to lead a more exciting life and express their emotions more freely they can quickly lose both their unhappiness and their excess pounds.

Research workers sometimes use the pulse rate as a guide to the level of bodily metabolism. When the heart beats quickly, either as a result of exercise, a feverish illness or emotional excitement, it's a sure sign that the body's furnaces are burning more brightly and consuming more fuel. Anything which inflames the emotions increases the rate at which we burn up calories. Film star Glenda Jackson loses weight whenever she is keyed up by her work. 'I went to Australia to do a play a year or two back and lost ten pounds in two weeks just from sheer stage-fright,' she reports. Taking a risk, falling in love, losing your temper, watching a rib-tickling film, plunging from the highest diving board at a swimming pool, or starting a new business venture can have the same effect. Anything that stimulates your pulse rate and steps up your output of stress hormones will increase the rate at which you burn up fat. Give a test subject an injection of 1 mg of adrenalin and his heat production will be temporarily increased by 20 per cent. Encourage him to lead a more outgoing emotional existence and his rate of metabolism will be permanently raised and with it his happiness, sense of fulfilment and zest for life.

● *Don't take drugs unless they're medically essential.* The person who drinks large quantities of alcohol puts on weight not only because he consumes too many liquid calories, but also because he's constantly imbibing a sedative drug which slows his metabolic processes and curbs the rate at which he burns up fuel. The same is true of people taking medically prescribed anti-histamine tablets, tranquillizers, sleeping pills and anti-depressants. A housewife becomes depressed because she has to perform the soul-destroying, unremitting chore of keeping her house neat and tidy, while her husband goes on exciting business jaunts round the world. Her doctor doses her with anti-depressant drugs. Three months later she feels lower than ever. Now, in addition to feeling fed up with her mundane housebound existence, she's also mortified by a sudden increase in weight and an equally rapid loss of energy. She feels sluggish and tubby. To raise her mood, and give herself a little false confidence, she starts to hit the cocktail trail. But this only accentuates her sluggishness and makes her fatter still. The answer to her problem lies not in the sedation of liquor and pills, but in the stimulus of emotional excitement and work fulfilment. People who are overweight, tired, depressed and anxious need to find themselves in action, rather than attempt to lose themselves in drugs.

● *Listen to the wisdom of the body.* If the appetite-regulating mechanism is to work effectively, it's necessary to eat slowly and listen to the cues that tell you when you've had enough. For many people, eating is more a habit than an urgent biological need. They eat because food is tantalizingly displayed before them, not because they're actually hungry. They tuck into a plateful of spaghetti bolognese not because their digestive juices are flowing and their mid-brains are crying out for sustenance, but because the clock tells them that it's time to eat. This is particularly true of people who are overweight, who are more readily stimulated to eat by external visual cues than by the signals emanating from within their own bodies.

This was neatly demonstrated by a series of experiments conducted by Professor Stanley Schachter of Columbia University. He took a group of volunteers, some fat, some slim, and got them to swallow a small balloon designed to record the hunger contractions occurring in their stomachs. With the aid of this device he found that the overweight subjects were relatively unresponsive to what was going on inside their stomachs. Whereas 70 per cent of the slim volunteers reported feeling a quickening of appetite when hunger pains gripped their stomachs; this was true of only 47 per cent of the fatties. For them it was more the sight of food, or the awareness of the passage of time, that encouraged them to eat.

This was demonstrated by another experiment in

which Professor Schachter invited people to take part in a test of 'autonomic reactivity', for which they had to be wired to instruments which recorded their heart rate and electrical skin resistance. This complicated arrangement was no more than a blind to conceal the fact that the real purpose of the test was to determine whether or not the volunteer's rate of eating was affected by their estimation of the passage of time. For half an hour they were left alone while their responses were supposedly being monitored. Then the experimenters returned to the test room casually nibbling a biscuit. Handing the guinea pigs the tin of biscuits, they invited them to help themselves while they filled up a personality questionnaire. Exactly half an hour later the researchers returned to the test room. Unbeknown to the volunteers, the clock placed conspicuously before them had been doctored to run either fast or slow. In some cases it showed that the experimenters had been away from the room for only twenty minutes, in others for as long as an hour. This made little difference to the slim subjects, but obese individuals showed definite evidence of eating by the clock. When they thought an hour had elapsed they consumed twice as many biscuits as they did when the faked clock indicated the passage of only twenty minutes.

In addition to not knowing when to start eating, most obese people find it difficult to tell when to stop. In many cases they gobble their food so quickly that they don't give their bodies time to know when they've had enough. It takes at least twenty minutes for food to be absorbed and messages to be transmitted from the stomach to the brain's satiety centres. During this time a good trencherman can consume a thousand calories and add another few grams of fat to his already spreading belly and thighs. Food must be consumed slowly if the appestat is to be given a

137

chance to work effectively. Inveterate gobblers must train themselves to eat more slowly. They should develop the habit of savouring each mouthful of food and chewing it until it has attained a liquid consistency. This will improve their digestion and increase their enjoyment of food. If slowing down proves difficult, practise putting down your knife and fork between each mouthful of food or try handicapping yourself by holding your knife in the wrong hand. In this way you'll rediscover the sheer sensual delight of eating and give your mid-brain a fairer chance to keep your weight under proper control.

Individuals who tend to put on weight must also overcome the desire to be good boys and girls by always licking their platters clean. Far too many unwanted calories are consumed by following this thrifty habit. Has it ever occurred to you that most of the food we eat each day – including biscuits, butter, bread and beer – is not fattening? If you're an average male you probably need about 2,300 calories a day to keep yourself in energy balance. If you're a woman the daily ration is likely to be nearer to 2,000 calories. Whatever you eat up to this point merely supplies your basic metabolic needs and cannot possibly make you fat. It's the food consumed beyond this limit that does the damage. You'll avoid consuming these unwanted calories if you eat slowly and listen carefully to the 'switch-off' signals from the mid-brain. This will mean that sometimes you will have to leave food uneaten on your plate. You may think this an insult to the cook, or an appalling waste of expensive fodder, but food is more surely wasted when it's allowed to go to fat than when it's quietly given to the dog.

If the appestat is to control our weight accurately and automatically, we must listen to the wisdom of the body and eat only when we're hungry and stop the moment that we've had enough. This adds enormously to the gastronomic delight of eating, especially when sufficient exercise is taken to generate a really healthy appetite.

It is said that Dionysius the Greek tyrant once complained bitterly that he was not enjoying the black broth placed before him. 'I do not wonder,' said his chef, 'for the seasoning is wanted.' 'What seasoning?' asked the tyrant. 'Running, sweating, fatigue, hunger and thirst; these are the ingredients with which we season our food,' replied the cook.

Follow the dynamogenic programme and you'll lose your surplus weight without sacrificing your love of delicious food.

7

Affairs of the Heart

It's rare to find Andalusian peasants suffering from angina, Masai warriors burdened with high blood pressure, or Watutsi tribesmen dropping down dead from sudden heart attacks. These are primarily the diseases of affluence. Now that we have licked the diseases of indigence (tuberculosis, malaria, smallpox and cholera), we are left to suffer the problems of indolence. Chief among these is coronary disease, which is now by far the commonest killer of middle-aged men in all the major industrial nations. In Britain nearly one in three businessmen fail to live long enough to collect their well-earned pensions – their premature deaths being generally due to cardiovascular disease.

Studies reveal that this insidious killer has its onset at a remarkably early age. Tests conducted by the University of Saskatchewan show that the cardiovascular efficiency of Canadians reaches its peak at about the age of twelve, and from that point onwards slowly declines. By the age of twenty the majority of Western men show some evidence of heart disease. When post-mortem examinations were performed on three thousand victims of the Korean war, it was found that half the American soldiers below the age of thirty had already developed mild damage of their coronary arteries, while a further quarter showed evidence of advanced heart disease. Similar results were obtained when post-crash autopsies were performed on four hundred Royal Air Force pilots. Again a surprisingly high incidence of incipient heart disease was revealed. Even among these seemingly fit young men evidence of severe cardiovascular disease was found in 30 per cent, and of milder degenerative changes in another 45 per cent. This means that whatever side of the Atlantic you happen to live on, if you're a man over the age of twenty, you have no more than a one-in-four chance of having a healthy heart. Your prospects are better if you're a woman, although statistics show that with the growing use of the contraceptive pill and the increased consumption of cigarettes, more women than ever before are suffering heart attacks. What is responsible for this modern epidemic? Why are so many people maimed, or stricken dead in the prime of their lives by angina, hypertension and coronary disease?

The answer to these questions is complex. There are several factors known to predispose to heart disease, such as obesity, high blood pressure, smoking, raised blood cholesterol level, stress and lack of exercise. Heredity also plays a part. If your father, mother and grandfather died of a heart attack before they reached pensionable age you can be fairly sure that you have inherited an above-average risk of contracting heart disease. But there's no need to adopt an air of resignation and sit back and wait until you're locked in King Coronary's suffocating embrace. You can greatly increase your chances of survival by losing excess weight, giving up smoking, maintaining a check on your blood pressure, keeping relaxed and, above all else, stepping up your level of physical activity.

Surveys show that people who lead active lives considerably reduce their risk of coronary disease. One of the earliest of these studies, conducted by the Medical Research Council in 1949, investigated the health records of the men who operate the London buses. It compared the incidence of heart disease among the drivers, whose work was purely sedentary, with that of the conductors who, while collecting fares on a double-decker bus, walk 8.5 kilometres (5½ miles) a day and climb a height equivalent to that of a small mountain. Analysis revealed that the drivers suffered more than twice as many rapidly fatal heart attacks as their more active mates. It might be

141

argued that the drivers, as well as leading less active lives, also had to cope with the strain of piloting a fifteen-tonne bus through crowded London streets. Stress rather than inactivity could have been the cause of their untimely deaths. To test this theory the Medical Council's research team embarked on another study. This time they directed their attention to Post Office employees, and made a comparison between the health records of men who had sedentary jobs with those who were engaged on postal delivery rounds. This showed the same link between coronary disease and physical inactivity. Post Office clerks, it was found, suffer twice as many sudden fatal heart attacks as postmen, whose work involves walking constantly from door to door and climbing endless flights of stairs.

Since these early reports were published many other epidemiological studies have been made, all of which confirm that hypokinesis, or lack of activity, is a prime cause of heart disease. In the famous Framingham community study, conducted by the United States Public Heart Service, a group of over 5,000 citizens living in the Massachusetts town of Framingham were subjected to a detailed medical examination and then closely monitored for the next ten years for signs of heart disease. As a result of this detailed prospective study it was found that coronary disease developed almost twice as frequently among men who defined their activity status as 'mostly sedentary' as in those who had described themselves as being 'moderately active'.

Why should this be? What beneficial effect does the heart derive from regular activity? The answer to this question is five-fold:

1. Exercise increases the mechanical efficiency of the heart.
The heart is only an elaborate muscular pump and, like every other muscle in the body needs regular exercise to keep it in trim. Two thousand years ago Hippocrates

propounded the 'Law of Use' which states: 'That which is used develops. That which is not used wastes away.' This is as true for the cardiac musculature as it is for the muscles of the legs and chest. The heart is a masterpiece of mechanical engineering. Although it weighs no more than 0.5 kilos (1 lb), this tiny muscular sac achieves the remarkable feat of circulating more than 9000 litres (2000 gallons) of blood a day. And it keeps up this prodigious work output for as long as we live, being relatively unfatiguable and also amazingly adaptable. If you're a clerk, and lead an habitually idle life, your heart will be small and relatively underpowered. If you're a stevedore your heart will grow big and strong and possess a correspondingly higher work capacity. Because of its greater development, the heart of a long-distance runner or cross-country skier may weigh twice the average and be capable of pumping 40 litres (70 pints) of blood a minute instead of the customary 25 litres (44 pints). This gives a greater reserve of power in cases of emergency, or when sprinting up a flight of stairs or chasing after a bus. It also explains the lower pulse rate of the trained athlete. Since the well-developed heart has a greater stroke output, it doesn't need to beat so often to circulate a given volume of blood. The resting pulse rate of a fit individual is often twenty beats a minute less than average. This greatly eases the burden on the heart, resulting in a saving of up to thirty thousand heartbeats a day. It also provides the heart with longer periods of rest, and improves the circulation to the cardiac muscle, which only takes place during the diastolic or resting phase of the heart's cycle. In this way the fit heart is better adapted both for activity and for rest. It is equally prepared for the circulatory demands of mountain climbing and idling in a fireside chair when, because of its superior efficiency, it does half to two-thirds less work than the untrained heart.

2. Exercise improves the coronary circulation.

Anginal pain and heart attacks arise when the coronary blood vessels become narrowed by fatty deposits or blocked by blood clots. This restricts the supply of blood to the actively contracting heart muscle and can result in ischaemic pain (angina), sudden failure of cardiac muscle function (heart attack) or death of sections of cardiac muscle tissue (myocardial infarct). At rest about .25 ccs of blood flow through the network of blood vessels supplying the heart walls. When we indulge in violent exercise this gentle stream becomes a rushing torrent, possibly sixty times as great. This makes it extremely difficult for clots to form, or for fatty deposits to accumulate in the walls of the coronary blood vessels. The risk of clot formation is always greatest when we're at rest, which explains why patients recovering from an operation are always encouraged to resume their normal activities as quickly as possible. It's not the rolling stones that gather moss, nor is it the actively working hearts that become silted up with fatty deposits.

Exercise also helps to expand the coronary blood vessels. Whenever a muscle is used certain chemicals called metabolites are released into the bloodstream as a by-product of muscle metabolism. These metabolites have the immediate effect of dilating the intra-muscular blood vessels, and so augmenting the blood flow according to the muscle's increased circulatory demands. This applies to the muscles of the heart as well as to those of the arms, legs and trunk. Exercise also has a more permanent effect on the intimate circulation to the heart. Post-mortem studies show that the coronary arteries of the average sedentary Western male become increasingly narrowed with the passage of time. But this is not an inevitable concomitant of the ageing process. The narrowing of the coronary arteries is not due to physiological ageing but to a pathological process of disuse, atrophy and decay. Keep your heart in vigorous use and your coronary circulation will remain as ample at fifty as it was at twenty-five, if not actually better. Dr George Mann of

144

the Vanderbilt University, Tennessee, proved this latter possibility when he studied the hearts of a group of Masai warriors, aged between fifteen and fifty. Throughout their lives these tall, well-built men walk 19 kilometres (12 miles) a day tending their herds of goats, sheep and hump-backed Zebu cattle. As a result of this constant vigorous activity their hearts keep free of degenerative disease. In fact Dr Mann discovered that under the daily stimulus of high levels of physical activity their coronary arteries actually *increased* in size with each passing decade. This makes them far less prone, if not totally immune, to coronary disease.

Experience shows that regular exercise, as well as being the finest prophylactic against cardiac disease, is also one of the most effective ways of recovering from a heart attack. Tests on laboratory dogs given an experimental blockage of a coronary artery show that the animals recover more quickly when they are put through a regimen of vigorous physical exercise. This provides the spur which enables them to compensate for their artificially-induced disability. The more actively their hearts are made to work, the more metabolites are produced within their cardiac muscle. This added chemical stimulus coaxes their remaining healthy coronary blood-vessels to dilate, and promotes the forging of new anastomotic links between the various branches of the vascular tree, which helps to bypass the experimental blockage. The same consideration almost certainly applies to human victims of natural heart attack. In 1967 Dr Terence Kavanagh, medical director of the Toronto Rehabilitation Center, instigated a programme of exercise therapy for seven hundred patients recovering from heart attacks. Eight years later he conducted a follow-up study to see how they had fared. This showed that only a fraction more than 1 per cent had had further problems with their hearts, compared with the 6 to 12 per cent relapse rate found among coronary patients who had not been given any systematic form of exercise.

All too often patients who have had a heart attack are beguiled into leading an over-protective life of idleness and ease. This is the worst thing they could do. To strengthen their hearts and overcome their disablity they must be courageous enough to lead an active life (though, of course, they must progress in easy stages). This also applies to patients suffering from anginal pain. In 1818 the famous British physician William Heberden recounted the tale of a patient with angina who 'nearly cured' himself of his chest pains by spending half an hour a day sawing logs of wood. Few doctors at the time followed this lead, or risked encouraging their cardiac patients to stop regarding themselves as invalids and start to resume a normal life. But a century and a half later a group of doctors from the Mayo Clinic in Rochester, Minnesota, carried out a trial of exercise therapy in the management of angina. At the end of a year of progressive exercise therapy, five of the eight patients they studied had lost all their anginal symptoms, while the remaining three had experienced a marked lessening of the frequency and severity of their painful spasms.

But why wait for illness to strike? The correct time to start taking exercise is before the heart becomes diseased, particularly since in 40 per cent of cases the first symptom of cardiac illness is sudden death. For these unfortunate individuals tomorrow is too late to adopt the dynamogenic way of life.

3. Exercise reduces the tendency of the blood to form clots.
Laboratory experiments show that physical activity facilitates the process of fibrinolysis – the natural mechanism by which the body breaks down the mesh of fibrin filaments which form the warp and weft of blood clots. This is of major prophylactic value in the prevention of clots, whether of the heart, lungs, brain or legs. But to have this beneficial influence the exercise must be tough.

To determine just how much activity needs to be

taken, the National Heart Institute of America tested a small group of youthful volunteers on a treadmill, measuring their oxygen consumption to assess their work-rate, and analyzing samples of their blood to determine variations in the tendency of their blood to form clots. These tests showed that mild exercise like walking makes no difference whatsoever to the blood's clotting power, whereas brisker exercise, such as jogging for a minimum of five to ten minutes, produces a noticeable increase in fibrinolytic activity. The maximum effect, however, is only derived by running flat out, or taking part in vigorous exercise which is likely to produce fatigue if maintained for five or more minutes. This brings about a marked fall in the tendency of the blood to form clots – an effect which can last for an hour or more after the exercise stops. For this reason violent exercise is now advocated by the National Heart Institute as a valuable form of fibrinolytic therapy. As such it rivals, and is in many ways far superior to, the anticoagulant drugs such as warfarin and heparin which are widely used in medical practice to prevent thrombus formation. These drugs can give rise to internal bleeding and sensitivity reactions severe enough to warrant the carrying of a warning card, whereas the side effects of vigorous exercise, such as weight control, increased vigour, heightened sexuality and greater stamina, are wholly beneficial.

4. Exercise reduces the blood pressure.
The major effort employed by the heart is devoted to driving the blood around the body's 60,000-mile arterial circuit. The higher the blood pressure, the harder the heart has to work. This helps to explain why people with a raised blood pressure have four times the normal risk of succumbing to heart attacks. But then hypertensive (high blood pressure) subjects are also more prone to develop strokes, hardening of the arteries, retinal haemorrhages and kidney failure. Theirs is a common cause of prema-

ture death. In fact it's been estimated that if all forms of cancer were eliminated the expectation of life of the average forty-year-old male would be increased by only two years, whereas he could gain a four-year extension of life if even moderately high blood pressure were eradicated. There is reason to believe that the adoption of a dynamogenic lifestyle would go some way towards achieving this goal. High blood pressure is largely a product of our high tension/low vitality way of life. It is favoured by such things as smoking, a diet low in roughage but rich in salt and animal fats, and three factors which are closely related to our hypokinetic life style – unresolved tension, obesity and lack of physical exercise.

The blood pressure of people under stress is invariably raised, and rightly so, for this is part of the body's normal defence mechanism. Whenever we're in a dangerous situation we need to have the blood coursing through our arteries preparing the body for the primitive responses of flight or fight. Providing these pressure surges are short-lived they cause few problems, for even the relatively thin-walled arteries of the brain can withstand blood pressures ten to twenty times the normal resting level. Difficulties arise largely when the blood pressure levels remain elevated for long periods, which can lead to permanent damage to the arterial walls. This frequently happens today when stress is induced by situations rather than by events, and is not rapidly relieved by purposeful activity. Meeting a leopard in the primeval forest caused a short-lived elevation of blood pressure which was quickly dissipated by picking up a club and beating the beast to death or, more probably, running hell for leather to the safety of the nearest cave. Driving a car through difficult traffic conditions today can cause an elevation of blood pressure which is sometimes double the resting level and which can persist for hours on end. Struggling through a financial crisis at work, suffering a constant battle of wills with a recalcitrant teenage child, or living in a state of constant marital discord, can cause blood pressure levels to soar and remain elevated for months on end. This can be relieved by taking some form of vigorous abreactive exercise. If you can't take it out on your colleagues at work, take it out on your opponents on the tennis court. If you're too Spock-trained to get stuck into disciplining your children, get stuck into taming your garden instead. Whenever you feel the pressures of life mounting, lift the lid off the emotional pressure cooker by indulging in some form of vigorous activity. This will enable you to let off steam and help you keep your blood pressure down to reasonable proportions.

Regular exercise, by controlling your weight, will also lessen your risk of developing hypertension. People who are fat normally have higher blood pressures than those who are slim. This is easily explained, for the heart and blood vessels operate rather like a domestic central heating system. The more radiators there are installed in the house, and the more complicated the system of interconnecting pipes, the higher the resistance in the circuit, and the greater the work that has to be done by the circulating pump. The same applies to our internal vascular plumbing. Every pound of fat we lay down is equivalent to installing another radiator in a central heating system, and increases the length of the arterial circuit by approximately one mile. This adds to the workload on the heart, and leads to an inevitable elevation in blood pressure. If you're overweight at present, follow the dynamogenic programme outlined in this book and your weight will fall, taking with it your unhealthily raised blood pressure.

And if you're not the slightest bit overweight, but have a higher than average blood pressure, you can still benefit by embarking on a couse of vigorous exercise. Tests show that, in a way that is at present not wholly understood, regular exercise helps to keep the blood pressure at optimum levels. Dr John Boyer, of the Human Performance and Exercise Laboratory, San Diego, discovered this when he encouraged a group of hypertensive patients to follow a regimen of gentle jogging. Though they made no other changes in their way of life, this produced an average fall of over twelve points in their blood pressure within six months.

5. Exercise lowers the blood cholesterol levels.
In today's coronary drama, cholesterol stands out as one of the most notorious members of the *dramatis personae*. Invariably it is cast in the villain's role – a fatty interloper which stealthily enters the body in the rich foods we eat, and insinuates itself in the walls of the blood vessels, where it leaves behind a trail of fatty degeneration and decay. To bring this domestic tragedy to a halt, the interloper must be banished from the land by ridding the diet of cholesterol-rich foods. Breakfasts must be taken without bacon and eggs, bread spread with hydrogenized vegetable oil instead of natural butter, coffee drunk without milk, pork meat stripped of its delicious crackling and strawberries eaten without cream. But is this heroic abnegation really necessary? Is cholesterol really as toxic as the pedlars of soft margarines, vegetable cooking oils, low-fat yoghourts and lecithin granules suggest? The answer to these questions is a vehement and resounding 'no'! Cholesterol is vital for the maintenance of bodily health. It plays an essential part in the repair of damaged lining membranes, is a vital ingredient in the manufacture of the sex hormones and bile acids, and an indispensable constituent of many body tissues, notably the brain, nerve cells and adrenal glands. To meet these constant needs a certain amount of cholesterol is extracted from the food we eat, but far more is synthesized within the body itself by the liver cells. Normally a careful balance is maintained, which ensures that the body receives an adequate supply of cholesterol without permitting an excess to circulate in the bloodstream and settle in the blood vessel walls. This is achieved by regulating the rate of cholesterol absorption, synthesis,

utilization and excretion. This enables races like the Eskimos to exist on diets rich in fatty meats without suffering an increase in either their blood cholesterol levels or their tendency to develop coronary disease. When diets are rich in animal fats the body automatically cuts down the rate of cholesterol absorption, and decreases the amount of cholesterol manufactured within the liver.

There is no doubt that stringent dieting can help to lower an abnormally raised blood cholesterol level, but this is treating a symptom rather than tackling the underlying cause of hypercholesterolaemia. The more fundamental question to be solved is why so many people in the Western world suffer an increase in their blood cholesterol levels, despite possessing an intrinsic regulatory mechanism which should control such untoward excesses. Possibly the strain of modern life plays a part, for tests show an elevation of blood fats whenever individuals are under stress, appear on television, pilot a plane, drive a fast car, work long hours, or go through the agonies of marital discord. Accountants, for example, show a steady increase in their blood cholesterol levels when they approach the end of the fiscal year and are under severe pressure which may necessitate the working of a seventy-hour week. During this time they make no changes in their diet, eat no more dairy foods or animal fats, and yet their cholesterol levels steadily mount as the financial deadline approaches. This increase is in no way related to their consumption of cholesterol-rich foods, but is closely paralleled by their personal assessment of the amount of strain under which they are working. More dramatic still is the rise in cholesterol levels which occurs when they go through the strain of marital disruption or divorce. Tests show that these domestic crises can cause a doubling of their resting blood cholesterol levels.

But cholesterol is only one of the many fats circulating in the bloodstream. It is the most talked about largely because it is the simplest to detect and measure. Others, such as the free fatty acids and triglycerides, are less stable and less easy for the biochemist to isolate and quantify, but play an equally important part in the production of cardiovascular disease. These too are poured out in increased quantities whenever we're under stress. One function of the stress hormones is to mobilize the body's fat reserves and release into the bloodstream an increased supply of fat globules. These provide a rich and ready source of energy should we need to run for our lives away from a bull, grapple with a mugger or break our way out of a burning building. This is an automatic, biological response to stress for which these days there's generally little call.

The dramas of modern life rarely call for strenuous physical activity. 'Flight or fight' might have been our forebears' natural response to danger, but it plays little part in the way we cope with adversity. The accountant, when he goes through the emotional traumas of divorce, has more need of a good lawyer than powerful muscles and a fuel-packed bloodstream. In the same way the life of a racing driver, piloting his Formula One car at speed round a perilous hairpin bend, depends more on the grip on his tyres than on the biochemistry of his blood. Stop for a moment and think of all the situations in your life that cause you stress. Do any of them require you to take hard physical exercise? You're in conflict with your daughter who insists on coming home late and keeping dubious company. You can't think how you're going to make ends meet or find the money to pay for your annual holiday. You're worried sick about losing your job. You're anxious about the energy crisis, the rising incidence of crime, galloping inflation, environmental pollution, drug abuse, high taxes, low moral standards, or the risk of nuclear war. Any, or all, of these circumstances may make your muscles tense, your blood pressure soar and your blood turn a shade paler from its increased content of fat. You're prepared for fight or flight, but neither action is appropriate. Inflation is not an entity you can fight, and there's nowhere in the world you can flee to escape the threat of nuclear war. So you remain tense, with a dangerously elevated blood pressure and a bloodstream supercharged with fats which are likely to be deposited in your blood vessel walls. This makes you a prime candidate for a heart attack. For this contemporary dilemma there's only one sensible solution, and it's not to give up eating butter and eggs! If you can't escape the stress of modern life, you can at least indulge in some form of vigorous exercise that will dissipate its physiological effects. This will work off your muscle tensions, lower your blood pressure and burn up the excess fats that are circulating in your blood.

At one time it was held to be impossible to reverse the ravages of arterial decay. Once fatty plaques had been deposited in the blood vessel walls it was believed that nothing could be done to shift them. Now it is known that damaged arteries can undergo a process of spontaneous recovery providing conditions are favourable for their repair. Reduce the lipid loading of the bloodstream and the fatty sludge lining the blood vessel walls will be slowly reabsorbed. This was first demonstrated by Dr David Blankenhorn of the University of California, Los Angeles. He took X-rays of the legs of a number of patients with high blood cholesterol levels, after first injecting a radio-opaque dye into their bloodstream. In twenty-five cases he discovered definite signs of arterial disease and fatty deposits causing narrowing of the blood vessels. These people he placed on a cholesterol-lowering diet, combined with a daily dose of anti-cholesterol pills. After twelve months on this programme he took further arteriograms of their legs and found evidence of spontaneous regression of the atheromatous narrowing of their blood vessels in 36 per cent of cases. It is likely that the same, or possibly better, results could have been obtained by introducing these individuals to the pleasures of regular fat-dispersing exercise, instead of placing them on a joyless regimen of pills and stringent dieting.

For a long time it was not understood why some people could have a raised blood cholesterol level and yet show no apparent increase in their tendency to develop cardiovascular disease. The mystery was eventually solved by two British doctors. Working independently, Dr G. J. Miller of the Medical Research Council, Penarth, Wales, and Dr N.E. Hiller of the Department of Cardiology, Edinburgh, showed that there are two basic kinds of cholesterol, one of which tends to favour the formation of arterial disease and the other to keep it at bay. Cholesterol, they discovered, does not travel in the bloodstream in isolation, but in combination with substances called lipoproteins. These fall into two main categories – high density lipoproteins (HDLs) and low density lipoproteins (LDLs). Through their experiments the two British doctors revealed that it is the cholesterol attached to LDLs that tends to be deposited in the blood vessel walls, while cholesterol attached to HDLs is automatically routed to the liver for excretion. They also discovered that people who are overweight, or who live on a diet rich in animal fats, are liable to have high levels of LDLs in their bloodstreams. This makes them prone to heart disease. Those with a preponderance of circulating HDLs, on the other hand, are relatively immune from cardiovascular disease. Certain individuals are fortunate in that they are born with a predisposition to maintain high levels of protective HDLs. Until they reach the menopause, women are also blessed with a high level of circulating HDLs, which must go a long way towards explaining their much-reduced incidence of coronary disease during childbearing years. But what can be done to help middle-aged men whose forebears have passed on the tendency to generate the wrong kind of cholesterol? Is there no way in which they can step up their output of HDLs and so keep their blood vessels clear of fatty deposits? Strangely enough they can take a useful step in this direction by having the odd glass of wine or can of beer, since moderate consumption of alcohol helps to boost the output of HDLs. This no doubt explains why autopsies on chronic alcoholics show them to have rotten livers, but generally remarkably clean, unblocked arteries.

Another way of increasing the output of HDLs is to take plenty of vigorous exercise. Over the years hundreds of London businessmen have kept themselves fit by visiting Al Murray's famous City Gym. More recently, this well-equipped gymnasium has been the centre of biochemical research carried out under the auspices of the Sports Council. This has shown that middle-aged men who take part in a planned programme of conditioning exercises not only look better and feel better, but also show an increase in the quantity of HDLs circulating in their blood, and a corresponding reduction in their levels of serum cholesterol, triglycerides and free fatty acids. These beneficial changes can be observed within a few weeks of commencing training, and persist as long as the exercises are maintained. Research carried out at Stanford University, California, by an English *émigré* physician, Dr Peter Wood, shows that regular joggers also have an unusually high level of HDLs in their blood. As he reports, 'The runners have a blood picture that might be mistaken for that of young women – a group in which heart disease is rather rare.'

Even brisk walking helps to raise the level of HDLs and flush the arteries free of their deposits of cholesterol. This was demonstrated at the Universiy of Minnesota's Laboratory of Physiological Hygiene, when a group of overweight young men was given a sixteen-week programme of progressive exercise on a treadmill. To begin with they were asked to walk for no more than fifteen minutes a day at a leisurely pace of only 2–4 km/h (1·5 mph). Later they were encouraged to walk both further and faster, until eventually they were walking at just over 4.8 km/h (3 mph) five days a week for ninety minutes a day. At the end of this four-month conditioning course their stamina had improved, they'd lost more than 5 kilos each in weight, and they showed an average 16 per cent increase in the levels of HDLs circulating in their blood. In this short time they had changed from being prime candidates for the coronary club, to having a much-reduced chance of succumbing to premature heart disease.

In these five ways exercise benefits the heart – by increasing the mechanical efficiency of the heart, improving the coronary circulation, decreasing the tendency of the blood to form clots, lowering the blood pressure and reducing the level of fats circulating in the blood. No other measure can do so much to further the health of the heart and reduce the cruel toll of coronary disease. Medicines may be found which counteract hypertension, and others which lower blood cholesterol levels, or reduce the clotting power of the blood, but no one drug performs all these functions at one and the same time as does exercise, or without the slightest risk of side effects.

In the prevention of coronary disease the arguments are all in favour of the dynamogenic way of life. Yet curiously enough many people refrain from taking strenuous exercise because they fear it might provoke a heart attack. They steer clear of sports halls because they recall one or two dramatic press accounts of middle-aged men dropping down dead while playing squash. Their excuse for not putting on a pair of track shoes and joining the hordes of joggers in the park is that a friend of a friend of a well-informed source told them the story of a fifty-year-old advertising executive who had a massive heart attack when he first donned a track suit and took a gentle plod around the block. And if that's pure hearsay, they remember clearly the two-thousand-year-old legend of Pheidippides, the heroic Greek soldier who ran back the 40 kilometres (26 miles) to Athens carrying the news of his countryman's victory at the Battle of Marathon, only to collapse and die from exertion at the gates of the city. Graphic tales like these suggest that whenever people get the feeling that they want to take some form of strenuous exercise, they ought to take Mark Twain's advice and lie down until the feeling passes away. But is there any substance behind these cautionary tales? Is there any way in which vigorous activity can damage the heart?

This question was discussed at the 1970 meeting of the World Congress of Sports Medicine, the unanimous verdict of the world's experts being that physical exercise alone is not a killer, unless it is superimposed on some pre-existing disease, or is taken by an unfit individual. Dr Alfons Kereszty of Budapest reported three cases in which top-class athletes – a footballer, a boxer and a wrestler – had all died suddenly while participating in their chosen sports. But each of these athletes had had a previous history of coronary disease and might as easily have had a heart attack in his sleep or while climbing a flight of stairs. Dr James Moncur of Scotland told delegates that during the previous year sixty-four Scots had died while taking part in sport, mainly as a result of accidents or from using faulty equipment. Only twelve deaths had resulted from a heart attack and the majority of these had occurred while golfing, fishing or playing bowls – pursuits which are considerably less strenuous than many everyday activities such as hurrying down the street to catch a bus. By the sheer law of averages some people will die while they are exercising, just as some will inevitably have a heart attack when they are having lunch. But this is no reason for giving up eating or for shunning exercise.

Providing certain simple precautions are taken, it's possible to indulge in vigorous activity without the slightest risk of damaging the heart. This has been proved by the practical experience of conditioning centres throughout the world. Dr Thomas Cureton has supervized the fitness training of thousands of middle-aged businessmen at the University of Illinois Physical Fitness Center. The routine he employs is tough, involving three or four one-hour work-outs a week of vigorous activity, calisthenic exercises, squat jumps, chin-ups, jogging and swimming. And he reports, 'If vigorous exercise of this type could precipitate a coronary attack, we would have a good many, but we have never had one.' When the Fitness Center celebrated its twentieth birthday Dr Cureton was able to report that fifty thousand men had passed through his hands without a single mishap. Dr Kenneth Cooper has also attested to the safety of the programmes of exercise employed at his Aerobics Activity Center in Dallas. Since its inception in 1971 somewhere in the region of six thousand people have trained under Dr Cooper's eagle eye. None have come to harm. As the guru of the world's band of happy hoofers says, 'On our tracks alone, we have recorded over one million miles of running and jogging without a single fatality.' Further confirmation of the innocuous nature of aerobic exercise comes from Dr Malcolm Carruthers, who maintained a careful five-year study of two thousand 'healthy' people attending Murray's City Gym. During this time not one suffered a heart attack – a clear indication of the prophylactic value of regular exercise. The experience of the coronary patients undergoing rehabilitatory exercise therapy at the City Gym was equally encouraging. An actuary would have expected several of them to have had further heart attacks in the course of Dr Carruthers' five-year study. In fact only one suffered this fate, and he was a lukewarm member who made only sporadic visits to the club. His death occurred at home several days after his last work-out, and was more closely related to his dilatoriness than to his over-exertion in the gym.

By an overwhelming margin the evidence shows that strenuous activity, far from damaging the heart, is essential for its continuing health and functional efficiency. But the exercise needs to be chosen with care and pursued with caution. If you follow the first step of the dynamogenic programme, outlined in the final chapter of this book, you'll get your full ration of cardiovascular exercise (see page 235). But do observe the following precautionary rules:

1. Get fit first

Don't start a course of vigorous physical exercise if you know you're sadly out of condition. If you're more than 20 per cent overweight, lighten the load on your heart by shedding a few pounds before you start playing squash or going for a daily jog. If you're a heavy smoker, take the precaution of cutting down your consumption of cigarettes before you embark on any form of fitness training. Better still, give them up completely.

If you have any doubts about your health consult a doctor before you start your activity programme. This is particularly advisable if you're a middle-aged male more used to handling a pen than wielding a tennis racquet. Preliminary medical check-ups are essential if you suffer from high blood pressure, poorly controlled diabetes or any form of heart disease. Providing you're reasonably fit your doctor may give you the go-ahead to exercise after briefly listening to your heart, measuring your blood pressure and monitoring your pulse. Other physicians may request an electrocardiogram (ECG), which records the electrical activity of the heart and provides a useful indication of the functional efficiency of the heart muscle. Although ECGs are not foolproof, and fail to show up many cases of established coronary disease, they have a definite predictive value. A five-year study of 18,000 civil servants working in the centre of London showed that men who have an abnormal ECG have a five times greater than average risk of dying from heart disease. More valuable information still can be obtained by subjecting the heart to 'stress testing'. This involves taking an ECG while the test subject is walking on a treadmill or riding a static bicycle. Under the strain of this additional loading it's often possible to spot minor cardiac irregularities, brought on by an insufficient coronary blood supply, which would otherwise remain undetected. This is a warning sign that under the stress of strenuous exertion the individual may be prone to have a heart attack or develop anginal pain. 'Stress testing' appears a sensible screening measure to adopt even if it involves no more than examining a person's pulse rate and heart after he's climbed several times up and down a chair. Nobody in his right mind would buy a secondhand car before subjecting it to an exhaustive road test, and it seems equally rash to pass a heart fit for vigorous use when it's only been examined under resting conditions. In America there are now scores of medical centres offering stress ECGs for fitness enthusiasts. In Britain these can only be obtained at a handful of centres when they are specifically requested by a cardiologist or general practitioner.

2. Start gradually

Harm arises when people who haven't exercised for years try to recapture their youth and lost vitality in a sudden flutter of vigorous activity. Hearts which have done no more than flutter gently during a Hitchcock movie may be mortified if they are suddenly made to pound away on a tennis court. Calf muscles which for years have only been gently flexed on the foot controls of a car may get bitter and twisted if they are brought out of retirement and abruptly used to climb a mountain. Necks which have been constantly fixed over a desk may be put out if they're suddenly twisted in a judo hold.

We are very much creatures of habit and object strongly to any violent change in routine. So the vital switch from a routine, sedentary existence to a vibrant, dynamogenic lifestyle needs to be made gradually. To obviate the risk of strain, follow the schedule of limbering exercises charted on pages 273–6 before you take up, or resume, any form of unaccustomed activity. And break yourself in gradually. If you aim eventually to keep yourself in trim by swimming twenty lengths of a pool, be content to swim no more than two or three lengths on your first outing, then gradually increase the distances as your fitness improves. And if your target is to jog 5 kilometres (3 miles) a day, start out by striding the distance, then add the occasional trot. Make sure you can walk before you attempt to run. Remember that the aim of cardiovascular conditioning programmes is to train, not to strain.

3. Choose a suitable time

Individual idiosyncrasy determines the ideal time to exercise. Some people are slow starters and find it difficult to exercise first thing in the morning. They're happier to take their sport at the end of the day when they're more alert. Others prefer to blow away the early morning cobwebs and get the day off to a good start by going for an early-morning jog or swim.

People with a tendency to run to fat may find it useful to reserve their most vigorous activities for the lunch hour. This will help to burn up fat and also to assuage their midday hunger pangs. Those with stressful jobs can benefit by taking their exercise at the end of the working day. This can be an excellent way of working off the tensions of the day, and is as potent a tranquillizer as a glass or two of scotch. But never indulge in *vigorous* exercise within an hour and a half of taking a meal, for during this time blood is shunted away from the heart and muscles to the actively working abdominal organs. And avoid strenuous exercise when you have a chest infection or heavy cold. Under these conditions you're unlikely to derive either enjoyment or worthwhile benefit from your endeavours, and it's just possible that you may provoke a spread of infection to the membranes surrounding the heart – a serious conditions known as bacterial pericarditis.

Once you've found the ideal time to take your cardiovascular conditioning exercise, stick to it. Make it as much a part of your daily routine as brushing your teeth.

4. Warm up first and cool down afterwards

Most people realize the value of gently loosening up their muscles before they participate in violent sport. But few realize that these preliminary warming-up exercises also help to improve the circulation to the heart and so lessen the risk of sudden heart attacks. Generally speaking the lower an individual's fitness status, the more time he should devote to warming-up. Many people make the mistake of thinking that warming-up exercises are strictly for the sporting elite. But if Sebastian Coe needs a ten-minute warm-up before he enters a race, the ordinary weekend runner needs to spend not less time but more. And don't feel self-conscious about performing a set of calisthenic exercises at the tennis club before you go on court. If you're a grey-haired grandparent of three, you may think it looks a trifle ostentatious to be cavorting about on the baseline before each game, jogging on the spot, toe-touching and flinging your arms from side to side. But it's much less dramatic to start the game in this way than risk ending it ten minutes later by being helped off court with a slipped disc or pulled hamstring. Besides, you didn't mind limbering up when you were young and agile; why should it bug you now when you're not so young and far less agile and so more urgently in need of the loosening up bends and stretches?

Be equally careful to end each spell of exercise with a gentle cooling down period of two to three minutes. This gives the circulation a chance to settle down gradually to its resting state. After a hectic game of squash never collapse exhausted in the changing room, but gently wind down by slowly packing away your gear, taking a shower and having a brisk rub-down. Similarly after an energetic jog round the park don't try suddenly to switch off your engines from full steam ahead to stop. Instead gear down by doing a final lap of honour at a steady walking pace. This will maintain the circulation to your heart and brain, and stop the blood stagnating in the dilated arteries of your legs and the flushed capillaries of your skin. The importance of this precautionary measure was demonstrated some years ago when a hundred men were exercised to the point of exhaustion on a treadmill, and then asked to stand stock still. Seventeen of the volunteers promptly fainted. Deprived of the chance of slowly readjusting the distribution of their blood, they had failed to maintain an adequate circulation to their brains and so collapsed. Mishaps like this can be prevented by paying as much attention to the post-exercise cooling down period as to the preliminary warm-up.

5. Avoid static exercises

At one time it was fashionable to indulge in isometric exercises – a form of movement which increases the tension in a muscle without making any alteration in its length. Businessmen were assured that they could improve their health without clambering out of their chairs, providing they tensed their leg muscles occasionally by pressing their feet against the ground, and tensed their biceps by gripping their desks and trying to lift them from the floor. This schedule of exercise was tailor-made for sedentary souls who didn't like to venture into the great outdoors, or run the risk of disturbing their carefully coiffured hair. But while isometric exercises undoubtedly help to maintain muscle tone, they are of little help in keeping slim and do nothing to improve the function of the lungs. What's more, they promote tension rather than relaxation and can be positively lethal for the heart. When natural exercises are taken, such as running, swimming, dancing and cycling, the beating of the heart becomes both faster and stronger. This increased cardiac output would make the blood pressure soar, were it not for the fact that rhythmical exercise has the additional effect of dilating the peripheral blood vessels. This decreases the resistance in the arterial circuit, with the result that in practice there is very little change in blood pressure when rhythmical exercise is taken. But when isometric exercise is taken there is no chance for the peripheral arteries to relax. In fact, the more firmly the muscles are tensed, the more they squeeze down on the intramuscular blood vessels. This increases the resistance to the flow of blood and inevitably makes the blood pressure soar. For this reason isometric exercises are not suitable for people suffering from hypertension or any form of heart disease.

6. Work hard

Experience shows that you won't get fit playing tiddly winks or Snakes and Ladders. You've got to work hard to benefit your heart and lungs. Ten years ago the Medical Rescarch Council studied the leisure activities of 17,000 executive grade civil servants and then kept a close watch on the men's subsequent medical histories. They discovered that the men who were active at the weekends had about a third of the risk of developing coronary disease as those who remained idle. But to provide this prophylactic benefit the exercise had to be of 'high intensity', and had to be continued for at least fifteen minutes. Hearts were safeguarded by swimming, tennis, brisk walking, climbing five hundred or more stairs, and by heavy gardening, and not by more gentle pursuits such as golf, painting, paper-hanging, polishing the car or hoeing the garden. Confirmation of this finding came when Dr Ralph Paffenbarger, of the Stanford University School of Medicine, studied a total of 17,000 students of Harvard University and found that only those who took part in intense physical exercise for a minimum of three hours a week improved the function of their hearts. This involved burning up at least two thousand calories a week in vigorous activity. Anything less strenuous produces no noticeable benefit for the heart.

Recent tests show that to condition the heart it's necessary to exercise vigorously for at least twenty to thirty minutes, three times a week. During these exercise periods the heart needs to be worked continuously at about three-quarters of its full capacity. The safest way of achieving this is by monitoring your pulse rate. To find the optimum level at which to exercise, subtract your age from 200, and then subtract a further 40 to 20 points depending on your estimate of your standard of fitness. This will give you a rough guide to the maximum pulse rate you should maintain while carrying out your thrice-weekly stint of cardiovascular conditioning. Thus if you're a fit thirty-year-old you should aim to push your pulse rate up to around the 150-beats-a-minute mark while exercising. Whereas if you're a sadly out of condition forty-five-year-old, your target level of training should force your heart to beat at no more than 115 beats a minute. In this way you'll condition your heart both safely and effectively.

7. Keep in training

If you want to maintain the health and efficiency of your heart you can't afford to rest on your laurels. It's possible to improve the functional efficiency of your heart within six weeks of embarking on a cardiovascular conditioning course of exercise, but it's equally possible to lose all these benefits in the next six weeks if you allow yourself to slip back into a state of idleness. To keep alive and alert, adopt the dynamogenic programme outlined in detail in the final chapter of this book and stick to it for the rest of your life.

8

The Dynamics of Success

Nothing succeeds like success, and nothing works like work. Without purposeful action you'll do nothing, achieve nothing and be nothing. Sustained effort is the secret of success in life, love, politics, business and war. As Emerson said, 'The world belongs to the energetic.'

Failures are not made, they arise by default. The Pulitzer Prize-winning author James Michener, whose books have sold over fifty million copies and been translated into more than fifty languages, discovered this lesson early in his career. Born into poverty, he was forced to work from an early age. By the time he was eleven he was supplementing the family income by getting up at four in the morning to deliver papers, seven days a week. At fourteen, while his widowed mother filled her day with sweatshop sewing, James worked a ten-hour day as an apprentice plumber. This early experience might have given him a lifelong antipathy to work; instead it instilled in him the conviction that hard work was the open sesame to every worthwhile achievement. This view was reinforced some years later when economic circumstances forced his family to part and he was placed for a while in a local workhouse. Here he made friends with many of the elderly inmates. Listening with fascination to their life histories, he concluded that the factor which had contributed most to their failure was an inability to work hard and purposefully. This realization gave him a life-long respect for work, which enabled him to become one of the world's most successful authors. As he recalled in his seventies, 'From this workhouse experience I generated a positive reverence for work. I saw it as the principal means whereby people achieve what they want and avoid what they don't want.'

Many youngsters today find it difficult to share Michener's credo. Some are highly critical of their parents' allegiance to the Protestant work ethic. They look around them and can only view work as a demoralizing chore. They fail to see that the fault lies not with the activity itself, but with the use to which it is put. Work need not be the bane of man's existence. When properly applied it can be satisfying, fulfilling and ennobling.

Economists estimate that fully 80 per cent of Americans are under-employed. No wonder boredom is one of the ailments of the age. How can people feel fulfilled when their lives are neither full with purpose nor filled with action? No wonder the world is beset with so many under-achievers, when vast numbers of people are content to fritter away their days in numbed idleness. People today are frustrated, bored, dissatisfied and discontented simply because they lead lives which are excessively dull and sedentary.

That is a fate that could never befall the dynamogenic leading lady of *Auntie Mame*. 'Live! Live! Live!' was her constant rallying cry. Mame knew the secret of vitality and always despised those individuals who led humdrum, mediocre existences and were too idle to reach out and grasp the riches that life has to offer. 'Life is a banquet,' she cried, 'and most of you suckers are starving to death.' But few heed her warning. Pampered and distracted by the candyfloss of modern life, most people fail to achieve their full potential. In our ignorance, we even encourage our children to follow the same drab, hypokinetic lifestyle. In their infancy we teach them to sit still, suppress their natural curiosity, accept what they are told, and keep a firm rein on their emotions. If they show any signs of originality or adventurousness we push them firmly back into line. If they express a passion for collecting butterflies, making model trains, studying the stars or scribbling poetry we tell them not to waste their time on frivolous pursuits. If they reveal signs of

167

youthful exuberance we diagnose them as being 'hyperactive' and sedate them with drugs so they're easier for parents and teachers to handle.

We expect our children to dress in school uniforms, sit passively for hours on end in school desks and lead during term-time an orderly, nine-to-four existence. Yet this is a time of their lives when they should be most playful, curious and adventurous. In forcing them into the strait-jacket of passive conformity at so early an age we stifle their initiative, drive and spontaneity. How different the lives of the young of most other species. We expect lambs to gambol, bear cubs to romp and fight, kittens to indulge their explorative urge and young chimps to tease and test the authority of their elders. We recognize that these activities are an essential part of growing up, and an important testing ground on which immature animals can assess their capabilities and prepare themselves for the challenges that lie ahead. Yet we deny this vital training to our young. We do not encourage them to be energetic, hardy, courageous and innovative. All that we ask is that they should apply themselves to their school books and attain a reasonable level of academic achievement. Yet countless sociological studies have shown that success in life does not depend on the possession of a high I.Q.

Sir William Galton, the world famous eugenicist, believed that there were three prerequisites for high achievement – a modicum of ability, zeal and a capacity for hard work. Thousands of people have the ability to succeed, but very few combine with it the necessary strength of motivation and the willingness to work relentlessly until they achieve their goal. An analysis of history's most prodigious talents shows that even genius is the product more of persistence than percipience. It's a quality which folklore claims is compounded of one part inspiration and ninety-nine parts perspiration. Major scientific discoveries don't just happen. They are invariably the result of hours of painstaking, and often frustrating, labour. First there is a long incubation period during which the problem is pondered from every conceivable angle and all relevant facts and possible solutions reviewed. This may be followed by a moment of sudden inspiration when a novel idea presents itself seemingly without effort or premeditation. But this is not the end of the creative process, for the new theory still has to be tested and developed. To the outsider the act of creation often means only the momentary flash of inspiration when the shadowy is made plain – the dramatic instant when Newton, lying under the apple tree, became abruptly aware of the full implications of gravity, or when Archimedes, lying idly in his bath, was suddenly brought face to face with the laws of hydrodynamics. But in focusing on these exciting bursts of creativity, we overlook the hours of inquiry which were their necessary antecedents and sequels. Without this painstaking but unspectacular endeavour Einstein would not have been able to conceptualize his theory of relativity, or Galileo develop the astronomical telescope and lay the foundation of the modern scientific method. It took Copernicus thirty years of painstaking research before he had developed his theory of the solar system to a point where he felt ready to publish his seminal work *De revolutionibus orbium coelestium*. And Darwin, after reading a text by the Reverend Thomas Malthus, which inspired him to conceive his species theory, spent over twenty years cross-checking his data and developing his ideas, until he reached the point when he could publish *The Origin of Species*. This is the stuff of greatness. As William Hogarth, the eminent eighteenth-century painter, said, 'I know of no such thing as genius, genius is nothing but labour and diligence.'

We succeed, less by luck and the inheritance of favourable genes, than by the application of labour and diligence. The more we do, the more we are. This is particularly true in the world of commerce. Tests show that the tsars of industry are invariably made rather than born (unless they happen to be Henry Ford II or Paul Getty Junior). When publisher Michael Korda studied the lives of high-flying executives for his book *Success!*, he discovered that the single most important factor leading to business success was high vitality. To get on in the world of commerce you've got to have energy and drive. You need the industry to get things done, to overcome the obstacles in your way, to achieve your goals and move from one post to the next. And it's fascinating to note that this inner dynamism, as well as helping you live off the fat of the land, will also help to keep you among the slimmest in the land. Top businessmen, for all their affluence and expense account lunches, tend to be svelte, not stout. A survey of high-earning American executives published some while ago in the *New York Times* showed that only nine per cent of them were more than ten pounds overweight. You can't be a dynamogenic character and put on weight.

The world's most successful military commanders have also been men of outstanding vitality. They've required a good tactical brain and a shrewd understanding of the men they command, but above all else they've needed the courage and will to *act*, for wars are won on battlefields, not on the flag-strewn maps of base camp tacticians. For a leader to do the right thing in battle is commendable; to do the wrong thing is regrettable; to do nothing is unforgivable. As General Sherman said, 'Better action without much knowledge than much knowledge and feeble action.'

It is by our individual enterprise that we gain success and by our personal achievements that we attain status. People are honoured for what they do, not for what they have. Few people today honour the memory of Prince Nicholas Esterhazy, the wealthy eighteenth-century nobleman, who rebuilt the Schloss Esterhazy in such elegant renaissance style that is was known as the Hungarian Versailles. Yet many continue to revere the man who was for thirty years his palace guest and protegé, Franz Joseph Haydn. The temporary kudos of the one man rested on his material riches, the lasting reputation of the other on his masterly work. We are remembered not for the social position we hold, but for the things we do – even if we haven't done them! Thus William Tell is remembered for the apple he never shot, Paul Revere for the ride he never made, and King Alfred for the cakes he never burned. However many PR consultants he might have employed, Hitler would always have gone down in history as a malign demagogue because his deeds were evil. To protect our reputations we do not require the services of professional image-builders, but the will to act in the way we would wish to be remembered. If we want to be brave we must act courageously, if we want to be found convivial we must spread good cheer, if we want to be trusted we must act with honesty. In this way we become the person we want to be.

Providing we have sufficient motivation and the willingness to work hard and consistently, few things are beyond our grasp. As the poet Ella Wheeler Wilcox has said, 'If you are seeking health, wealth, usefulness, skill in any direction, there is nothing and no one who can hinder your attainment of the coveted boon, if you are willing to work and wait.' Having such a quest gives life its purpose and zest. It's the shortest road to stardom, the quickest cure for boredom and the most certain recipe for happiness. Life can never be dull for people who are working hard to achieve their chosen goal. William Makepeace Thackeray lived his life at an incredible pace. At one time he was writing novels and also contributing regularly to six different newspapers. Deadlines loomed up at him like flagpoles in a downhill skiing race. But far from turning himself into a writing machine, or making himself a hermit in his study, he still found time to gamble, stand unsuccessfully for parliament, carouse, go to fashionable parties and frequent all the Bohemian cafés and drinking places. Though he worked prolifically, he could still chuckle, 'I wallow in turtle and swim in claret and Shampang.'

The same applied to Franz Schubert. Few composers can rival Schubert's creative output. During his brief lifespan of thirty-one years (in those days even the hardiest, most vital individuals couldn't withstand the ravages of typhoid fever) he created more than a thousand works, including symphonies, operas, piano sonatas, string quartets and songs. In one incredibly fecund year he wrote four operas, two symphonies, nearly 150 songs and numerous ancillary chamber and choral works. Yet this intensity of work didn't detract one iota from his lusty enjoyment of life. Dynamogenic individuals like Schubert aren't crabbed and narrow in their interests, but exuberant participants in life's exotic carnival. Schubert lived life to the full. Rising at six, he would devote the morning to composing, have lunch and then spend the remainder of the day socializing with his friends. In the afternoon they might ramble through the Viennese woods. After supper they would often repair to the nearest hostelry for a stein or two of beer, then back to one of their homes where Schubert would improvize on the piano, and friends recite their latest verse. Throughout his brief life Schubert was poor, but exceedingly happy. Friends recognized in him the 'divine spark' which illumined his work and enlightened his life.

Dynamogenic characters have a voracious appetite for life and achieve a monumental output by devoting themselves whole-heartedly to everything they endeavour. When they work they concentrate totally on the task in hand; when they play they give themselves over completely to spontaneous, unsophisticated merry-making; and when they unwind they relax utterly and completely. In this way, they sample the delights of life's highways and byways, and enjoy the best of all possible worlds. They are total people. For them all attributes are positively correlated. In ardently seeking fulfilment, they make their own fortune, and create their own fun. They also invariably enjoy a rich and satisfying sex life.

It's a myth, promoted by many misguided Freudians, that to achieve success you've got to sublimate your sexual energies. In fact the founder of psychoanalysis held the diametrically opposed view. As Freud himself wrote, 'I have not gained the impression that sexual abstinence helps to bring about energetic and self-reliant men of action or original thinkers or bold emancipators and reformers. Far more often it goes to produce well-behaved weaklings who later become lost in the great mass of people that tends to follow, unwillingly, the leads given by strong individuals.' This is born out by a study of the lives of history's most creative characters.

Consider Rubens, the great Flemish painter. Like all truly dynamogenic characters, this giant among post-renaissance painters showed an awesome lust for life. Art historians claim that his artistic output has never been challenged, even by the longer-lived Picasso. His interests were catholic, his industry immense. He had a passion for knowledge and a burning desire to learn more about archaeology, physics and astronomy as well as subjects such as anatomy, morphology and physiognomy which had a more direct bearing on his work. His travels throughout Europe were extensive and for several years he acted as a diplomat for the Archduke Albert. To accomplish these prodigious feats he rose at four in the morning and laboured steadily throughout the day. But he still found ample time to dine with his friends, and every afternoon at five rode along the ramparts of Antwerp on his fine thoroughbred Spanish horse. Rubens also recognized in himself a certain 'paganism'. This is revealed in the soft eroticism of his paintings which show something of the warmth of the relationship that he shared with his first wife Isabella, and even more so with his sensuous second wife, Hélène Fourment, whom he married when she was only sixteen. She was the inspiration and model for many of his later paintings, such as *The Garden of Love* and *The Fur Coat*, some of which have been described as being 'on the edge of pornography'. She was his romantic passion or, as he confided to his son, 'the joy of my old age'.

A similar pattern can be traced in the life of Victor Hugo, the great French poet, lyricist, novelist and playwright. A great romantic, he believed that 'The object of modern art is not beauty but life'. A voracious reader and gifted mathematician, he was showered with honours by his fellow countrymen. For his political work as an elected member of the National Assembly he was made a peer of the French realm. For his plays and novels he was elected to the prestigious French Academy. His energy was outstanding. Even in his latter years his pen continued in constant spate, producing more books after his sixtieth birthday than most authors complete in a lifetime. But Hugo was no stuffed shirt. He loved both life and pretty ladies. In addition to his wife, who bore him a large family, he had a number of affairs, and a passionate liaison with his mistress Juliette Drouet, whom he wooed and won from a wealthy French prince and for fifty years maintained as his devoted and adoring lover. And when, at the age of eighty, he was caught by his grandson making love to a young laundress, the old man chuckled, 'That is what I call genius.' Hugo recognized that the stamp of a successful life lies in its breadth as well as its profundity. The secret of dynamogenic living is not to indulge in narrow specialism, but to reach out with open arms and embrace the world in all its rich variety – to work, to play, to learn, to love, to feel, to grow, to create, to explore. Life should be viewed not with a spy glass, but through a gigantic fish-eye lens.

Although we live in an age of specialization, there's much to be gained by being a polymath. If you've the talent to be a chemist you've also got the ability to be a poet, pianist or explorer. If you've established yourself as a teacher, you've also got the potential for being a writer, actor or politician. Why neglect these reservoirs of untapped talent? Why plough a solitary furrow, when acres of virgin soil remain untilled? We may place Albert Einstein in the pigeonhole reserved for eminent mathematicians and physicists, but his personal life was far richer than this. In addition to developing his unified field theories he also wrote poetry, loved sailing, carried on extensive correspondence with his friends, played Mozart melodies on the violin and cycled in the countryside near his Palm Springs home. Paderewski was not only a pianist/composer, but also prime minister of Poland. John Wesley, in addition to being an itinerant preacher, was a successful barefoot doctor and a popular writer. Although he travelled over 8000 kilometres (5000 miles) a year mainly on horseback, and preached sometimes as often as three times a day, he still found time during his lifetime to publish some two hundred books. Getting up at five in the morning to fill his day as full as possible, he said, 'I am always in a haste, but never in a hurry.'

For the person who seeks success, the maxim 'Don't have all your eggs in one basket' seems far more appropriate than the equally popular adage 'Don't have too many irons in the fire.' If history is any yardstick, it pays to plunge into the furnace of life every fire iron you possess. In this way you'll broaden your personality, increase your satisfaction, swell your enjoyment and maximize your chance of success. You'll also gain charisma, for dynamogenic individuals don't hold power – they radiate it. They express the *élan vital*, which gives them personal magnetism, warmth and charm.

Here are four specific ways in which you can latch on to this power:

- *Formulate clear-cut aims*. As the writer Lord Lytton put it, 'The man who succeeds above his fellows is the one who early in life clearly discerns his object and towards that object habitually directs his powers.' In short, you can spend all your life

175

scurrying about on the field, but you'll never score unless you've got a definite goal to aim for.

Management by objectives is by now a well-established business technique. Executives work more effectively if they are given definite targets to aim for. The same is almost certainly true at shop floor level. Management consultants in the past have cajoled employers into believing that if they introduce measures to increase the job satisfaction of their workers they will help to banish their frustration, and in the process secure a useful boost to production. But recent studies suggest that this is not true. Programmes of job enrichment may improve the contentment of a team of workers without necessarily increasing productivity. This was demonstrated in a recent test, supervised by industrial psychologists, in which four groups of workers were given the task of sorting computer cards. One group was subjected to the full job enrichment treatment, being told that they alone were responsible for their work, so that they had the freedom and flexibility to organize their own work flow. Another was set definite targets which were demanding but not unrealistic, being told exactly how many record cards they were expected to process each hour. A third group was provided with these goals together with the enrichment perks, while a fourth was given neither targets nor perks. At the end of a few days the output of each worker was measured, and they were asked to fill in a questionnaire to assess their feelings towards the work. As might be expected the fourth group of workers found little satisfaction in performing their humdrum task. Happiness was considerably greater in the other three groups, but despite this a significant increase in productivity was only found when workers were given a definite goal to strive for. Flowers, frills and job enrichment fancies may keep employees cheerful, but it takes a definite target to spur them on to higher productivity.

More people now accept the value of laying down corporate goals and work targets, but many still fail to appreciate the value of adopting the same practice in their own lives. Lacking a clear sense of direction they flounder about like rudderless ships, unable to make use of life's favourable winds and prevailing currents simply because they have no clear idea of the port to which they are bound. These people don't plan to fail – they fail to plan.

Goals must be clearly defined, and to be effective must fulfil three basic criteria – they must be personal, realistic and specific. Successful people set their own targets and travel at their own pace to achieve them. It's futile wasting energy striving to achieve the second-hand goals handed down by your parents, and pointless struggling to keep up with the Joneses, unless you genuinely want what the Joneses have got. It's equally futile to set your sights too high. If you want to become a world-class high jumper, and can currently achieve a leap of only 1·5 metres (5 ft), it would be unrealistic to set yourself the target of clearing 2·3 metres (7 ft) by the end of this year. That would invite almost certain failure. Far better to aim for 1·5 metres (5 ft) this year then try to add another 15 centimetres (6 in) during the following season. The more clear-cut the target, the greater your chance of attaining it. Holding vague ambitions is little better than having no intentions at all. It's useless to say 'I want to be famous,' unless you specify the particular field in which you are going to excel and are prepared to answer all the ancillary questions of how and when and why. Don't be content to say 'I want to become a well-known author,' without planning a definite step-by-step programme of activities to lead you to that goal, starting with today. If this is your ambition, make a plan to sit down before the day is out and write a letter to your local paper. That will take you one tiny step towards your ultimate dream. Next week aim to write a brief article for the parish magazine. Then enrol for a class in journalism. After that, offer to compile a regular column on gardening, fishing or cooking for a small circulation magazine. You may not get paid for your labour, but you will gain invaluable experience, and move one step nearer to your chosen objective. Success, you'll discover, is not a destination but a journey. People who follow its track add zest to their lives and discover a renewed sense of purpose.

Psychiatrists find that lack of adequate direction and drive is the root cause of many people's psychic malaise. As Jung said: 'About a third of my cases are not suffering from any clinically definable neurosis, but from the senselessness and aimlessness of their lives. I should not object if this were called the general neurosis of the age.'

● *Work with wholehearted dedication.* Having fixed a clear objective, all that remains is to labour steadily towards that end. The plums of life don't fall into your lap unless you shake the tree. All the great monuments to men's achievement – the pyramids, the Panama Canal, the Taj Mahal – stand as silent testimonies to man's capacity for hard work. They may be considered the wonders of the world, but they are no miracles. They are in each case the product of a master plan, backed by hours of unremitting toil. It's been estimated that Stonehenge took more than 18 million man hours of labour to construct, and must have occupied a large proportion of the population of Britain for years on end. To create a modern masterpiece requires equal perseverance and industry. We like to think that things come easily to people of outstanding ability, but this is rarely so. Constant repetition may facilitate their skill, but they still have to work hard to achieve their goals. Mohammed Ali, surely the most successful fighter of modern times, may have started out with a pugilist's physique and lightning reflexes, but he would not have reached his pre-eminence in the boxing world had he not been prepared to spend hours practising his technique and improving his ringcraft. In the words of Joe Martin, the policeman who recognized his potential as a boy and gave him his first boxing lessons, 'He was just an ordinary kid – a bit of a smart Aleck – but he worked harder than any of the hundreds of other kids I taught. And he refused to be discouraged. You knew he'd do anything necessary to get to the top.'

Most high achievers recognize the importance of hard work. Voltaire's motto was *'Toujours au travail'* (Always at work); Sir Walter Scott's watchword 'Never to be doing nothing'. Others have adopted the Royal Air Force slogan *'Per ardua ad astra'* (By hard work to the stars). It's common to attribute people's success to their luck, breeding, contacts or charm, but closer inspection generally reveals that their achievement is built on the bedrock of painstaking endeavour.

It's often believed that top salesmen get where they are because they have a cheerful, extroverted personality, combined with an unshakeable faith in their own ability. But recent tests show that their volume of sales is more closely related to the number of hours they work than to their psychological make-up. This was revealed when a group of nearly two hundred trainee salesmen were asked to complete standard questionnaires designed to measure their self-esteem and extroversion. They were then given the task of selling academic textbooks to university students. After three months their sales records were compared with their psychological profiles. This showed that their success as salesmen was in no way related to their personality, but was closely allied to the length of hours they worked and the number of calls they made. As the psychologists conducting the experiment were forced to conclude, the findings fully vindicated the old adage, 'There is no substitute for hard work.'

● *Have courage.* In an achievement-orientated society, failure stands out as a heinous crime. Because of this stigma people refrain from embarking on new ventures, not because they're afraid to try, but because they're afraid to fail. They hold back from asking for a salary rise in case their request is turned down. Young men hesitate to ask an attractive girl out on a dinner date in case their overtures are spurned. Businessmen fight shy of making an after-dinner speech for fear they'll make asses of themselves. Others long to take up painting, but never pluck up the nerve to put brush to canvas, in case their early daubs are not the artistic successes they would wish. Some would like to take part in local government but haven't the guts to put their names forward for fear they'll end up bottom of the poll. These people, by lacking the courage to risk failure, ensure that they can never win. By being unwilling to make the occasional mistake, they end up making nothing. But, as Montaigne said, 'Failure is not a crime, failure to attempt is.' We'll never achieve anything of note unless we're prepared to accept occasional setbacks, emotional upheavals, uncertainty, unpopularity, financial crises, physical hardships and embarrassment.

It takes courage as well as effort to succeed. This was shown in a study carried out by two psychologists at the University of Texas. They analysed the factors which contributed to the success of two groups of high achievers – the one composed of successful US scientists, the other of high-flying graduates of the University of Texas Business School. The four behavioural qualities they studied in these men were their desire to work hard and keep busy, their willingness to accept challenging tasks, their competitiveness, and their reaction to the criticisms of others. The results showed that in both groups the highest incomes were received by people who scored low in competitiveness, but who worked hard, thrived on challenge, and were not deterred by the opinion or adverse comments of their colleagues. Contrary to popular belief it's not scoring over others that matters, but having the grit and determination to score for yourself. It was these qualities of fortitude that characterized men like George Washington, who was willing to be stoned by an angry mob rather than sacrifice his principles, Thomas More who walked willingly to the scaffold rather than surrender his beliefs, and William Harvey who persevered with his unorthodox theories concerning the circulation of the blood even though he was ridiculed by his colleagues and abandoned by many of his patients. By making a resolute stand these men achieved their goals and also asserted their individuality, for it's only by the fearless assertion of our principles that we can establish our autonomy and maintain our personal integrity.

You don't know what you can do unless you try. And you don't know who you are unless you have the courage to be yourself.

● *Be persistent*. From the cradle to the grave we are reminded that Rome wasn't built in a day, great oaks are only felled by a repetition of little strokes, and that a constantly dripping tap will wear away the hardest stone. We absorb the message, but only rarely do we put it into practice. In our everyday life we look for instant success. If we can't get what we want quickly and painlessly we abandon the quest. But great achievements are rarely easily won. In 1932 Charles Darrow, an out-of-work salesman, sat down at his kitchen table and set out to design a game. Scribbling on a piece of oilcloth, and using cotton reels and thimbles as counters, he eventually hit upon the idea of a board game involving the buying and selling of property. During the next few evenings he played the game with his wife and neighbours, gradually reshaping the rules and modifying the layout of the board. Such was the success of these evenings that several friends asked Darrow for copies of the game, which he painstakingly made by hand. Then he took the bold step of having a few sets printed, one of which he sent to Parker Brothers, one of the world's leading manufacturers of card and table games. They considered the new invention, decided that it broke at least fifty of the criteria for successful table games, and promptly rejected it. At this point most people might have thrown in their hand, or half-heartedly hawked the game to one or two other manufacturers. But Darrow was so convinced he was on to a winner that he risked every cent he possessed on having another five thousand sets printed. These he sold to one or two New York stores. Slowly the popularity of the new game grew. Then, by chance, a set was bought by a close friend of the Parker family. Her report to them was so enthusiastic that they agreed to give the game another test. This time they decided to go ahead and market it. From that moment on neither Parker Brothers nor Charles Darrow looked back. Some may say that there was an element of luck in Darrow's success, but fortune would not have entered into the equation had he not had the courage and persistence to back his hunch. Monopoly, the game he devised, brought Parker Brothers a windfall of £120 million and left Darrow a multi-millionaire.

The success of Aristotle Onassis can also be attributed as much to his dogged determination as to his undoubted financial acumen. When he was a youngster he decided to make his fortune by importing oriental tobacco into Argentina. Shipping in a small quantity of the finest Turkish leaf, he began a tour of all the cigarette manufacturers in Buenos Aires. But none showed any interest. So he left them samples of the leaf and a copy of his trading card, in the hope that one or two would eventually place an order. None responded. Determined to make a breakthrough and clinch his first sale he picked as his principal target Juan Gaona, the managing director of the country's largest cigarette manufacturers. Each day he stood outside Gaona's office, looking at him sadly and reproachfully as he arrived for work. At other times he maintained his silent vigil outside the director's home. Eventually his stubbornness paid off. Gaona could stand the mysterious picketing no longer, and asked the youngster what he wanted. Onassis explained that he merely wanted to sell him high-grade oriental tobacco. The businessman was amused by his quiet determination and a few days later gave him an order for £2,500. In later life the Greek magnate looked back on the £150 commission he earned on this deal as the foundation of his immense fortune. But without his youthful persistence the transaction might never have been made.

The research chemists at May and Baker also discovered the virtue of persistence when they went through the painstaking testing of 692 sulphonamide compounds before finally discovering M & B 693, the world's first effective drug in the treatment of pneumonia.

If you know what you want in life you can nearly always get it, providing you're sufficiently dogged, daring and determined.

9

The Fountain of Youth

For generations man has sought the secret of perpetual youth. The Greeks tried to stave off senescence by eating mussels, crabs and snails. Wealthy Germans in the nineteenth century endeavoured to recapture their flagging spirits by visiting Graefenberg and taking the water cures offered by Vincent Priessnitz, a semi-illiterate Silesian peasant who rediscovered the value of cold water bathing, and in the process earned himself a fortune of over £50,000. When the popularity of this fad waned, jaded Europeans of all nationalities flocked to the *Kumyss* curative stations in the Russian steppes, to drink the fermented milk of pregnant mares, and inhale the excremental odours generated by the breeding stables. Since then rejuvenation seekers have experimented with galvanism, vitamin pills, monkey gland extracts, novocaine injections and Professor Niehans Cellular Therapy. Recently there was a vogue for drinking *muska voda* – the mineral-rich spring water of Kladanj, a remote village in Bosnia which, legend claims, promotes long life, health and amazing sexual potency. Currently the craze seems to be for eating ginseng, the wonderworking Oriental herb. But medical research has failed to discover any specific curative properties in these elixirs of youth. Geriatric research has proved that it's not necessary to drink cider vinegar or swallow megadoses of Vitamin E to live to a ripe old age. Healthy longevity is the birthright of every human being – an inheritance we all too often squander by our indolent, unhealthy lives.

The average mammal achieves a lifespan that is roughly seven and a half times its age at maturity. This suggests that man could reasonably expect to live to be

120, and many physiologists believe this to be well within our capabilities. Pavlov, the great Russian physiologist, held the view that everyone could and should live to be a hundred. The failure of so many people to do so, he said, was due to 'intemperance, lack of regularity, and their own criminal attitude towards their bodies.' At present we think of centenarians as being rare freaks of nature, but in fact many more exist than is generally imagined. A short while ago a sample of British people were asked to guess how many people over the age of a hundred were currently living in their country. Their estimate rarely exceeded fifty, whereas the true number of centenarians at the time was known to exceed eight hundred. Americans might be equally surprised to learn that a tally a few years ago showed that there were over 11,000 people over the age of a hundred receiving US social security benefits.

These people have no special secrets to explain their remarkable endurance. They don't take patent remedies, eat macrobiotic foods or sleep with their bodies facing magnetic north. But they do invariably lead lives that are full of activity and rich in purpose. This was clearly shown by a study conducted by two German professors of psychology. They wanted to discover why some people live longer than others, and to fathom this mystery painstakingly followed the lives and fortunes of two hundred senior citizens aged between sixty and seventy-five. At the end of fourteen years' detailed observation they analysed their results, and found that the main characteristic of the survivors was that they had a more positive, active approach to life. They were also more adaptable and had a strong feeling of being needed by others and of use to society. Another study of 124 German centenarians reached the same conclusion, showing that the outstanding feature of these veterans was their lively, vivacious temperaments. The people who live to a ripe age aren't genetic anomalies, but ordinary individuals who in their early years have acquired the habit of dynamogenic living. This has been confirmed by a detailed study of over five thousand American centenarians, which has shown 'that the people who survive are not "biological accidents" as has been claimed, but people who in their daily living have made exceptional adjustments to life situations.'

These evergreen senior citizens know how to live life to the full. Take the case of Khfaf Lasuria, a small, sprightly inhabitant of the Caucasian mountains of Southern Russia. At the time she was visited by American gerontologist, Dr Alexander Leaf, Khfaf was over 130. In view of her age he might have expected to find her closeted quietly in her room reclining on an invalid's couch. Instead he discovered her pottering about in her garden tending her chickens and pigs, surrounded by a group of lively youngsters. She greeted him with traditional Georgian warmth. Together they toasted each other's health, first in vodka and then in wine. Then, helped by an excellent memory, and spiced with great good humour, she reminisced about the past and talked about the present. She had worked at the local collective farm since its formation and had been the co-operative's champion tea-leaf picker when she was over a hundred years old. For two years she had been retired from full-time work, but she continued to maintain her independence and keep herself active in her home and garden. When she wanted to visit her relatives in a distant village, as she had done recently, she merely hopped on the local bus and travelled alone. She was old, but in no way decrepit.

In the same way when Dr David Davies, of London University's Unit of Gerontology, visited the old stagers of Vilcabamba in Ecuador, he found them 'Bright, alert and active', not broken down by senility and disease. They ate a light, largely vegetarian diet, but were otherwise not particularly abstemious in their habits. Many smoked cigarettes made from tobacco grown in their own gardens and drank anything from two to four cups of unrefined rum a day. One notable feature of their lives was that most continued to work until within a few days of their death, like José David, an agricultural labourer who was still hoeing in the fields at 142, an age verifiable by his baptismal certificate.

What keeps these people so remarkably fit? The answer lies largely in the dynamic quality of their lives. Few have any use for cars, often travelling long distances over hilly terrain by foot. This regular strenuous exercise contributes far more to cardiovascular fitness than the Westerner's occasional game of squash or jog around the park. Take the case of Kosta Kashig, another centenarian investigated by Dr Leaf on his Georgian study trip. He was a shepherd who tended a herd of goats on grassy slopes more than 1500 metres up the mountainside. To reach him, Dr Leaf and his companions had to set out at dawn and trek for six hours up slippery mountain paths which in places became so steep that they had to be climbed rather than walked. So arduous was the journey that two of the party had to turn back. Yet Kashig, at the age of 106, was constantly making this trip in what he claimed was half the time! Doing so enabled him to come alive and stay alive, for there's no doubt that regular strenuous exercise is the finest prescription for a long and healthy life. This is confirmed by Georgian cardiologist, Dr David Kaklashvili, who has carried out extensive testing of the heart and lungs of these perennial Russian patriarchs and reports, 'The constant physical activity improves cardiopulmonary function so that the oxygen supply to the heart muscle is much superior to that in city dwellers.'

The inhabitants of Vilcabamba and Caucasia expect to go on living and loving until the day they die. As one 117-year-old Caucasian peasant said, 'Youth normally extends up to the age of eighty. I was still young then.' Our expectations of life are different. We anticipate problems once we've passed our allotted span of three score and ten. At this period of our lives we expect our memory to fail, our speech to falter, our gait to grow unsteady and our interest in life to wane. Senior citizens are told to take life easily in case they pull a muscle, slip a disc or precipitate a heart attack. At that age, when they seek treatment for minor ailments, their problems are often dismissed as inevitable accompaniments of the ageing process. Doctors reassure them that they're really doing remarkably well – considering their age. So we come to live up to our expectations. The physical decrepitude and general uselessness of the elderly becomes a self-fulfilling prophecy.

Jean Rawlinson presented herself for osteopathic treatment at the age of sixty-three, suffering from a stiff neck, painful back and arthritic knee. Her husband, several years her senior, had died when she was in her early fifties, but had left her wealthy enough to enjoy a comfortable standard of living. Until her rheumatic pains overtook her she had been outstandingly fit and athletic. She had swum regularly, played tennis at least three times a week, maintained the large garden of her delightful country home with little outside help, and exercised her horse every day. Now those days were gone. She felt an old woman. Less than three years before she could work all day and dance all night; now it was as much as she could do to clamber out of bed in the morning and drag herself through the very minimum of daily chores. What had gone wrong?

Examination showed that she had slight arthritis in her neck and knees, and a moderate degree of degenerative change in her lumbar spine, but these minor problems would have been present three years before and in no way explained her sudden decline. Why had she aged so rapidly? To find the answer to this question she was quizzed about the watershed period of her life. What had happened three years ago? Had she had an accident? Had she been confined to bed with a serious illness? Had she at the time been under considerable emotional stress? Nothing relevant sprang to her mind. Then, when asked what it was that forced her to give up riding and tennis, she provided the clue to the entire dilemma. When she reached the age of sixty she had misguidedly accepted the advice of her friends to act her age and take life a little more sensibly. At sixty, they suggested, it wasn't safe for her to carry on riding, or being so athletic on the tennis court. Unwisely she followed their advice and completely gave up riding, tennis, and all other vigorous activities which she thought might strain her system. She started to act as convention told her a well-brought-up lady of sixty should behave.

And so she *became* like a conventional sixty-year-old lady – unadventurous, slow and stately in her movements and limited in her activities. Gradually her body modelled itself to its newly appointed role. Her knees, which had probably been injured in an early sporting accident, seized up from lack of proper use. Her neck, without regular exercise to keep it supple and strong, became as rigid as a dried-out plastic sponge. And the joints of her lumbar spine, lacking sufficient activity to keep them mobile, became as difficult to get started in the morning as a veteran car after months of idleness in a garage. The remedy was obvious. After a few manipulative treatments she was free of pain and able to move her joints as freely as before. After that it was back to her riding, gardening, tennis, swimming and dancing, plus any other activities that took her fancy. She was advised to ignore the well-meaning advice of her friends. Nothing but herself, and her self-imposed limitations, were likely to prevent her carrying on with her riding and tennis into her sixties, seventies and eighties. After all, in their mid-sixties Borotra was playing tennis for France, Francis Chichester was sailing single-handed around the world and Blondin, the French acrobat, was turning somersaults on stilts on a tightrope! And at sixty-five Goethe could ride a horse for sixty-four hours on end without dismounting.

Obviously our conventional attitude to ageing is sadly

out of touch with reality. We expect people to quit the drama of life at the end of the first act, not at the final curtain. Recently sociologists have even propounded a 'theory of disengagement', which suggests that it is natural for people to gradually relinquish their hold on life as they age. What nonsense! It is as natural for people to lose their zest for life at sixty as it is for a man to lose his libido when he enters the priesthood. Sixty is not a time for giving up, but a time for taking up. At this age Enoch begat Methuselah, the Emperor Vespasian began to create the Coliseum, Tolstoy learnt to ride a bicycle, Gandhi started a new campaign for Indian independence and Catherine the Great took a fresh lover. Think how much poorer the world would have been without the activities of these lively sexagenarians, and consider how much more banal would have been their own existences. Our contemporary attitude to ageing is unscientific, demeaning, wasteful and cruel. Anyone who follows a policy of disengagement as he grows older sentences himself to a life of premature decay. Like the player in the last act of Shakespeare's strange eventful history, he will end up in a state of mere oblivion, 'sans teeth, sans eyes, sans taste, sans everything.' But physiological fact and practical experience confirm that this is not man's inevitable fate. Some diminution of strength may be inevitable as we enter our seventies and eighties, but not as much as most people suppose. During his eightieth birthday party, Charles Atlas demonstrated his strength by tearing up telephone directories and at eighty-five, George Hackenschmidt, the former world wrestling champion, demonstrated his fitness and stamina by jumping fifty times over the back of a chair. As we age our libido shows a gradual decline, but again not as much as is popularly believed. A study of over a hundred elderly men showed that 34 per cent of the men over seventy and 65 per cent of the men under seventy were still sexually active, with two out of five of the octogenarians averaging at least ten copulations a year. These figures would have been more impressive still if allowance had been made for the fact that some of the men being studied were virgins and others, though potent, had no available partners. If properly cultivated there is no reason why sexuality should not persist throughout life. Certainly some centenarians have been known to father children.

Sophie Tucker was wrong when she announced that 'Life begins at Forty'. Dynamogenic living can begin at sixty, seventy or any other age you choose. Irrespective of our chronological age, we should strive to keep the fires of life burning until the very day we die. This is the only way to promote life, and the only acceptable way of prolonging life. Who in his right mind wants to endure the indignities of medicated survival? What is life if it can only be preserved by drugs, drip feeds and oxygen inhalations? The purpose of dynamogenics is to enable people to live until the day they die. To paraphrase Dylan Thomas, 'Old age should burn and rave at close of day.'

Consider Grandma Moses, the farmer's wife who took up painting at the age of seventy-eight and went on to become one of the world's most famous primitive painters. From the moment she developed that consuming passion until the day she died at the age of 101 her life was filled with both purpose and interest. Exhibitions of her work were held throughout the world, one in Moscow being attended by 100,000 people. In ten years one firm sold 35 million of her greetings cards. Copies of her original works, of which she painted 1,500 during her last twenty years, sold for £7,000 – an outstanding price at that time for an untutored, primitive painter. She was entertained at the White House, interviewed on television, and fêted wherever she went. After nearly eight decades as a hardworking but obscure farmer's wife, she had achieved worldwide acclaim as a painter. She had discovered a new vocation, and with it a new purpose and interest in life.

Take also the case of Ben Duggar who, when he reached the age of seventy, was compulsorily retired from his post as Professor of Botany at the University of Wisconsin. At this age he felt far too young to be thrown on the scrap heap. He was still an exceedingly active man in both body and mind. He played golf, took long walks, danced like a Comanche and went bowling at least once a week. He wasn't ready to quit. So he talked himself into a job as a consultant for Lederle Laboratories. The job they gave him was to analyse six thousand soil samples for possible therapeutic properties. He threw himself into this new task with enormous zest. For months nothing happened. Then he examined one of his culture flasks and found that it had sprouted a golden mould. With great excitement he extracted the active organism and found that it possessed powerful bactericidal properties. At the age of seventy-three this reject of the academic world had discovered auremycin, the world's first broad spectrum antibiotic. Later he continued his experiments and discovered other members of the tetracyclin family, which were to become medicine's greatest allies in the fight against infectious disease. In maintaining the usefulness of his personal life, Ben Duggar had made an epochal discovery that was to preserve the lives of thousands of his fellow men.

We accept that it's important to establish goals in the early stages of life, but ignore the equal importance of maintaining a driving sense of purpose in our latter years. One of the revealing features of the hardy Georgian centenarians is their continuing sense of purpose. They still fulfil a useful function in the community – cleaning the house, weeding the garden, picking tea, tending the crops, feeding poultry and caring for their grandchildren. Instead of being pushed to one side, as happens in most industrialized societies, they are revered for their experience and age. Above all else they feel needed. As a 113-year-old Caucasian said when visiting gerontologists asked him whether he would be helping to build the new house next door to his own, 'Of course, they can't do without me.'

This is the right way to regard the elderly. They should be held in esteem, not treated as second-class citizens. Though they may not be as nimble or vigorous as youngsters, they still have a valuable contribution to make to society, not least in their length of experience and accumulated wisdom. After all, at eighty-five Verdi composed his marvellous *Ave Maria*, *Stabat Mater* and *Te Deum*, at eighty Goethe finished *Faust*, and at ninety-eight Titian painted his famous picture of the Battle of Lepanto.

One of the things that has done most to harm the health and psychological welfare of senior citizens has been the introduction of a compulsory retirement age towards the end of the nineteenth century. Prior to this time people carried on working until they either chose to retire or felt they were no longer capable of efficiently pursuing their chosen occupations. With a fixed retirement age people are forced to cease work whether they wish to or not; whether they have come to the end of their productive lives or are still at the peak of their creativity; and irrespective of whether they have alternative work to go to, or are likely to be under-occupied for the remainder of their lives. Ageism is a form of social discrimination every bit as evil as sexism and racism. By this one act the lives of many people are cut abruptly short. As a spokesman for the Soviet Institute of Gerontology has said, 'Man could live longer if he were allowed to work longer.'

Historians generally attribute the instigation of a fixed retirement age to the German Chancellor Otto von Bismarck, who decided in 1884 that sixty-five was to be the age at which German social security pensions were to be paid. In fact it is wrong to blame Bismarck for the invention of this appalling piece of legislation. This cruel and senseless measure was first applied in Britain two years after the 1857 Northcote-Trevelyan report recommended that a fixed retirement age should be introduced in the British Civil Service 'to remove those too old for effective work'. The age was set at sixty-five because this was considered the time at which 'bodily and mental vigour begin to decline'. But the rule is so hopelessly arbitrary. In the Victorian era the health of many people might have been declining at the age of sixty-five, due partly to poor medical services, malnutrition and the ravages of the then unconquered infectious diseases such as tuberculosis. But this is far less true today. Besides, while some people nowadays may be past their prime at sixty-five, many others are still in the pink of health and have many years of valuable service to give. Why waste their talent, knowledge and undoubted skill? Why put them out to grass if they are anxious to remain in harness? Particularly when for some this act is tantamount to signing a death sentence.

Primitive races in the past devised other methods of dealing with their unwanted elderly, which are in some ways more humane. Old stagers in one South Sea Island community were forced to climb a tall coconut tree. Once they'd scrambled to the top the tree was given a vigorous shake. Those who managed to cling on were considered fit to survive; those who couldn't fell to the ground and met almost certain death. The ritual was callous, but had the merit of introducing an element of selectivity into the retirement procedure. Those who passed the gruesome test were judged strong enough to carry on working, while those who failed were given a swift and humane dispatch. We observe no similar screening process, dispensing with the services of the fit and the unfit alike at an age when most have years of active service left to give to the community.

In Kenya, less than a century ago, a different method was used for coping with burdensome elderly people. When they fell sick, or become decrepit, they were carried from their homesteads and left abandoned in the bush. If they were too frail to survive they fell prey to the hyenas; if they had the strength to struggle back to their huts they were given a renewed lease of life. We employ a similar policy with our old folk the moment they show any signs of becoming troublesome. When they start to be a debit entry on our social balance sheet, instead of the creditors they have been throughout their lives, we remove them from the security of their homes and place them in the wilderness of a geriatric home. But generally we give them no chance to prove their fitness to return home and resume their rightful place in society. Theirs is generally a one-way ticket to oblivion. The procedure seems infinitely more humane, and certainly far more costly, than the practice adopted by the Kenyan tribesmen, but the end result is little different. By committing our old folk to geriatric ghettoes we relinquish responsibility for their care and genteelly speed their end. Experience shows that within six months of being admitted to a geriatric nursing home the death rate of elderly people rises 10 to 24 per cent above that of their contemporaries of similar health status who are left in community care within familiar surroundings. Taken suddenly from their homes, stripped of their independence, their activities curtailed and their individuality suppressed, these abandoned senior citizens often slip into a rapid decline.

Psychological studies show that to keep alive in an old folks' home you need the same tough qualities that aid survival in a concentration camp or prison. Six years ago Morton A. Lieberman, a psychologist at the University of Chicago, studied the fate of a group of elderly people who were admitted to three homes for the aged in the Chicago area. The ages of the group, which numbered over eighty, ranged from sixty-three to ninety-one. Despite their advanced years all were in good physical and mental health at the time of their admissions. Nevertheless some of these displaced persons died within months of becoming institutionalized. Of those who survived, all but 30 per cent showed a marked deterioration in their condition within the first year of entering a home. Tests on the hardy third, who appeared to have survived the experience intact, showed that they were outstandingly active, autonomous, aggressive individuals who maintained a high level of self-esteem. With these strong drives and personality characteristics, they were better able to withstand the pressures of institutional life. But given these qualities they were surely well equipped to continue to support themselves in the mainstream of society. Why place these individuals in social quarantine when they are suffering from no physical or psychological disease? Why not harness their talents for the benefit of the entire community, rather than leave them merely to subserve their own survival?

In societies where an increasing proportion of the population is past retirement age we haven't the resources to support large numbers of dependent elderly people, particularly when so many of them are perfectly capable of fending for themselves. Nor can we afford to let so many of them develop into helpless, senescent imbeciles. Experience shows that many people exhibit a marked deterioration in their mental health when they are admitted into institutional care. Senility is a thing that is widely feared. Many people are apprehensive lest they should finish up at the end of their days forgetful, confused, rambling and maniacally incoherent. In fact this is a fate that few elderly people suffer. Surveys show that only about five per cent of the population develop organic deterioration of their brains as they grow older, and those that do often conspire to their own downfall by leading unhealthy, inactive, withdrawn lives. (A recent study, reported in the *International Journal of Social Psychiatry*, revealed that only 22 per cent of sufferers from senile dementia have outgoing personalities.)

Mental decay is not inevitable. Popular articles about the brain are fond of quoting the fact from the age of twenty-five onwards several thousand brain cells a day die and are never replaced. Nobody bothers to quote the origin of this particularly gloomy item of information. Before writing this chapter I took the trouble to trace the source of this data. It stems, I discovered, from a piece of rough and ready research carried out over sixty years ago, in which a comparison was made between the number of cells contained in the brain of a man who died at the age of forty and a man who died at eighty. On the basis of this scant sampling, backed up by the post-mortem examination of only a few other brains, the research workers estimated the inevitable daily brain cell loss of the whole of mankind! Given the wide individual variation in the anatomy of the human brain, extrapolations of this kind are laughable, were it not for the fact that they influence many people to believe that a steady deterioration of brain function is inevitable with the passage of time. In adopting this pessimistic outlook no recognition is taken of the achievements of men like the elder Cato, who started to study Greek at the age of eighty, or the Spanish philosopher George Santayana who, as he approached ninety, was still compiling books of profound intellectual thought. The minds of these men continued to work with precision and clarity, not because they were composed of particularly hardy nerve cells, but because their brains were kept in constant use.

Laboratory experiments have shown that when animals are maintained in a stimulating environment their brains develop. Under these conditions their nerve cells grow, their brains become heavier, and an increased number of synaptic connections are established between individual nerve cells. Conversely, when brain tissues are under-employed they suffer a process of disuse atrophy. Thus if one eye of an animal is artificially obscured, the nerve connections leading from this eye are gradually lost, while the pathways stemming from the other eye undergo compensatory enlargement. In time, the animal acquires hyperacuity of vision in the eye that's being constantly used and becomes functionally blind in the other. In the same way, it's likely that the brains of elderly people will succumb to a process of disuse atrophy if insufficient use is made of their intellectual capacities. As a committee of the World Health Organization concluded, after studying the mental health problems of the elderly, the finest prophylaxis against senile decay is 'independence and activity'. But then there's little novel in this idea. Over two thousand years ago Cicero arrived at exactly the same conclusion. 'Old men,' he said, 'retain their intellect well enough if only they keep their minds active and fully employed.'

One of the major causes of senile dementia is a declining circulation to the brain. This can be mitigated by adopting the dynamogenic way of life. A man is like a tree: he tends to die on top first. If the sap stops rising it's the crown of the tree that starts to fail. In the same way, if the blood stops circulating it's the cerebral function that's the first to suffer. (That's why we faint when we're in a state of shock, or when we take an excessively hot bath which shunts too much blood to the surface of the body.) Most people visualize the brain as a solid mass of grey matter. In fact it's 80 per cent water, more fluid even than the blood. If it's taken out and put on an anatomist's bench the brain collapses like an unset jelly. As the years proceed the body undergoes a steady process of dehydration. This affects the brain as well as the muscles, bones and skin, and accounts for the major loss of brain weight between the ages of thirty and ninety, when the mass of the average brain falls from 1360 grams (3 lb) to 1105 grams (2·7 lb). In the twilight of our lives it's more important than ever to keep the brain bathed in an energy-rich fluid medium.

Mental functions decline if the brain is supplied with insufficient oxygen. This is almost certainly a major reason for the failing memory shown by so many elderly people. It's estimated that the brain is capable of recording over a thousand billion items of information. Even a studious centenarian is unlikely to reach the storage limit of this incredible data bank. So the problem of memory is not one of information storage, but one primarily of data recall. This process can be facilitated by submitting the memory to regular use, and by getting sufficient exercise to ensure the proper distribution and oxygenation of the blood. Tests on elderly hospital patients have shown that significant improvements can be made in their short-term memory by getting them to breathe pure oxygen for two sessions of ninety minutes a day. Most people can achieve the same effect, without the need for hospitalization and expensive oxygen therapy, by performing breathing exercises and taking regular aerobic exercise. This is an integral part of the dynamogenic programme outlined in the final chapter of this book. Those who follow this way of life can add years to their life, and life to their years.

Here are four valuable habits to acquire:

● *Don't be unduly influenced by the passage of time.* Chronological age is an exceedingly poor guide to what you can or ought to do. People who've safeguarded their health may be fit to climb mountains in their eighties, while others who've grown fat and flabby through inactivity could be at risk mounting a flight of stairs at forty-five. Don't let the spectre of age deter you from doing the things you feel to be within your compass. Take the days as they come. If you've played regular tennis in your seventies there's no earthly reason why you shouldn't keep playing into your eighties or even later. If you've kept yourself fit in your sixties by daily jogging, there's no reason why you shouldn't carry on until you are a hundred, like Larry Lewis, the San Franciscan waiter, who celebrated his 105th birthday by going for his usual 11-kilometre (7-mile) jog, and then walking 8 kilometres (5 miles) to work.

Many of the changes observed in elderly folk are psychological rather than physiological. Senility sets in when you lose your zest for life, have no plans for the future, and feel you've nothing left to contribute to the community. It begins, not when you start drawing your pension, but when you start saying, 'I'm too old to do that.'

A person's chronological age is set by the calendar; his physiological age by his attitude of mind and general approach to life.

● *Get yourself fit, and refuse to allow yourself to become a martyr to sickness.* Once people pass the age of seventy it's common to blame their age for every affliction they suffer. What can you expect if they get out of breath climbing the stairs? 'It's anno domini,' their friends say, and often their doctors too. The fact that they smoke too much, are overweight, sadly out of condition and anaemic is barely taken into consideration. When they're plagued with backache, and look like a bent hairpin every time they get up from a chair their trouble is ascribed to 'fair wear and tear'. Little is done to help them because of their age, even though they could probably be restored to health by a short course of manipulation or physiotherapy treatment. Through neglect of this kind our senior citizens are allowed to become increasingly infirm. But age is neither a disease, nor an adequate explanation for disease. A study carried out by a working party of American doctors, led by gerontologist Richard Besdine of Harvard Medical School, revealed that 10 to 20 per cent of people diagnosed as suffering from senility were actually suffering from treatable diseases such as anaemia, hormonal imbalance, depression, kidney failure and vitamin deficiencies. Dismissing their symptoms as signs of advancing age denied them both the possibility of cure and the chance of resuming a full and active life. As you grow older, neither expect illness nor willingly accept illness.

The greatest deficiency among the elderly is not

one of vitamins, but one of exercise. And yet when we set out to establish community recreational programmes, we invariably provide facilities for the young, who require them least, and totally ignore the demands of the old, who need them most. All the more credit then to enlightened local authorities, like London's City of Westminster, which provide a wide range of activities for its senior citizens including old-time dancing, swimming, keep-fit classes, theatre trips, seaside excursions, handicraft courses and light assembly workshops.

Medical research shows that it's never too late to get yourself in better shape. Some years ago Russian doctors took a group of sixty-year-olds and for ten years put them through a weekly session of tough gymnastic exercises. At the end of the period they were re-tested and found to be fitter on every physiological measurement than they had been at sixty. A similar rehabilitation programme was instigated by Dr Herbert de Vries, exercise physiologist at the University of California. He took a group of men aged between fifty and eight-seven and put them through a regimen of carefully planned exercise. All showed gains in physical health and a welcome reduction in nervous tension. By the end of a year they recorded an average drop of nearly five per cent in their body fat, an increase of more than nine per cent in their maximum oxygen uptake, and a growth of over seven per cent in their arm strength.

These programmes show that by following the dynamogenic programme outlined in this book it's possible for seventy-year-olds to recapture some of the fitness and vigour they had when they were forty. This will also help them to counteract weakness, stiffness and loss of balance – the three common handicaps of advancing years which contribute so much to geriatric accidents, falls, and general lack of confidence.

● *Keep active and purposefully occupied*. Don't stop working unless you want to run the risk of dying of boredom. When doctors from Birmingham University carried out a survey of a thousand men aged between sixty-five and seventy they found that nine out of ten were fit to carry on with their jobs. Bringing work to an abrupt halt at this, or any other, age can remove life's *raison d'être*, and usher in sickness, depression and premature death. It's a question often of do or die. As Jeremy Taylor, the seventeenth-century prelate, said, 'Idleness is the death of a living man.' (With the traditional allocation of sex rôles, women were more fortunate than men. Their involvement in housework never ceased, which may help to explain why female centenarians outnumber males by six to one.)

If you have the choice, never retire unless you've got something better to do with your time. If you keep active you'll be too busy to notice the passage of time, and too preoccupied to feel miserable. This is the secret of perennial youth. A few years ago a Swiss pharmaceutical company made a survey of elderly workers in Britain, and found that they had over five hundred claimants for the title of Britain's oldest worker. 'We have been amazed,' the firm reported, 'at the number of men in their nineties still doing a full day's work.' Even more remarkable was the positive approach these old stagers had towards their occupations. This attitude was typified by the remarks made by a ninety-one-year-old from Ramsgate, Kent, who at the time of the study was still putting in a forty-hour week as a cleaner and decorator, 'Working stops you feeling miserable. I think work is the secret of happiness.' An equally positive view was expressed by a ninety-two-year-old widower from East Mitcham, Surrey, who was still running a blind-making business which had been founded many years before by his father. 'I love my work,' he said. 'Men die when they stop working.'

● *Enjoy life's pleasures to the full.* Long-lived people don't dwell in the past, but live avidly in the present and continue to look forward eagerly to the future. They're always anxious to listen and learn, experience and explore. They never stop growing. Pablo Casals, the world-famous cellist, was a typical example. When asked in his eighties why he contined to practise four or five hours a day, the Spanish maestro replied, 'Because I think I am making progress.' This is an attitude of mind which should be acquired in childhood. Geriatric medicine, properly considered, starts in the kindergarten.

One of the fundamental principles of all life extension programmes is to cultivate the art of living each day as if it were your last on earth. Don't try to conserve energy – spend it. Like love, the more energy you expend, the more you will have. Don't worry about burning the candle at both ends. If the flame looks like petering out, go out and get more wax.

You're old the moment you lose your interests, don't know what to do with your time, and are no longer fascinated by the rich pageantry of life. Conrad Hilton, founder of the world's most prestigious hotel chain, was a truly dynamogenic character and retained an insatiable curiosity in the world around him until the day he died. In his eighties he continued to attend his office every day, and confessed, 'I like the tumult of life. I like its problems, its ever-changing stresses.' Time never hangs heavily on the hands of people like this. There are never enough hours in the day to satisfy their needs and compelling interests. Bernhard Berenson, the world-famous art historian and critic, had an enormous zest for life. His permanent battle was against the clock, his constant longing was to have more time to pursue his work. When he was approaching ninety he said wistfully to a friend, 'I would willingly stand at street corners, hat in hand, asking passers-by to drop their unused minutes in it.'

People like this have learned the secret of survival. They live on to an advanced age, but die young – and happy.

10

Eros Liberated

Sexual love is one of life's richest rewards, and among the strongest motivators of human behaviour. Some of the world's greatest works of art, literature, poetry and music have been created under Cupid's sway. For love people have quit their jobs, bid farewell to their families, committed suicide, squandered their wealth, and even given up their thrones.

This 'divine passion', as Socrates called it, is a vital part of our lives, so much so that plans are afoot to provide astronauts with female companionship on their longer missions into space. According to a spokesman of the American National Aeronautics and Space Administration, the absence of normal heterosexual relationships could place intolerable stresses on crews engaged in space flights of a year or more's duration.

As Freud clearly revealed, sex plays an important part in ordering our day-to-day behaviour. From early childhood onwards, eroticism fills our fantasies, modifies our goals, and shapes our interpersonal relationships. Even during sleep our sex organs remain active. Approximately every ninety minutes during the night men get an erection, and at roughly equal intervals women develop vascular engorgement of their vaginas. In Victorian times it was customary to deny the strength and urgency of human sexuality. Now it is fashionable to subject every facet of the phenomenon to microscopic study and detailed debate. Today it seems impossible to scan a novel or magazine without reading some reference to swinging couples, vibrators, multiple orgasms or oral sex. The subject is now as much a topic of public discussion as politics, food prices and the weekly football results. When an American psychologist made a study of the erotic content of American books, newspapers, plays, television and radio, he found an increase of 250 per cent in the number of references to sex in the decade from 1950 to 1960. Since then there has been a steady increase in sexploitation. But have we benefited by removing the veil of senseless prudery? The substitution of the modern scientific voyeur for the Mrs Grundys of old appears to have done little to improve our psycho-sexual health. People still write to agony columns complaining of the unsatisfactory nature of their sex lives. Impotence and frigidity remain two of the commonest symptoms psychiatrists are called upon to treat. And sexual maladjustment persists as one of the major causes of marital discord, being the predominant symptom of sixty per cent of couples who attend Marriage Guidance Counselling sessions in Britain.

Sex today seems to be becoming increasingly boring, mechanical and impersonal. The vibrator is hailed as the passport to connubial bliss. Mates are selected by computer rather than by the mysterious process of sexual attraction. Now, instead of losing ourselves in the enjoyment of sex, we stand back and analyse it like a time and motion expert. Was it as good as before? How long did it last? Should the foreplay have been maintained a little longer? Did we achieve a simultaneous climax? Are we reaching the norm, or should we make love a little more frequently to reach the national average? How colourless, calculated and contrived! Like eating, sex is in danger of becoming a bland, packaged routine.

By comparison, how different the sex life of our forebears. Sex for them was not a monochrome xerox print, but a fresh and original action picture, painted in vivid colour with free and flowing brush strokes. For the Romans it was as much a cause for celebration as the ripening of the harvest and the re-awakening of Spring. They followed the cult of Dionysius and worshipped at the shrines of Venus and Cupid. At the Bacchanalian feasts the wine was heady, the dancing wild, the music thrilling, and the loving intense. Effigies of Priapus, the God with the Lilliputian body and the Brobdingnagian penis, were hung everywhere as talismans. Fastened to the gateways of Roman cities as good luck charms, these priapic symbols often bore beneath them the inscription *Hic Habitat Felicitas* (Happiness Dwells Here). This was not the obsessional, neurotic sex of today, but glorious, untrammelled eroticism.

The same freedom and exuberance is to be found in the sexual behaviour of most native races. The early visitors to the South Sea Islands were captivated by the beauty of the Polynesian girls and also by their totally liberated, unselfconscious sexuality. When Captain Cook arrived at Tahiti on the *Endeavour*, he was met by a welcoming band of dusky maidens. With laughing eyes and flashing smiles they swam out to the ship and greeted the sailors with gaiety and passion. For Cook's travel-weary men the girls, with their lithe brown bodies glistening seductively in the tropical sun, provided an early glimpse of paradise. Paul Gauguin, the French artist, was also totally captivated by the beauty of the South Sea Islands and the sexual permissiveness of its vivacious inhabitants. Once he had discovered the simplicity and freedom of the Tahitian culture, he never again returned to the restrictive conformity of his Parisian home. Over the years some of this spontaneity has been lost. With the arrival of proselytizing missionaries, the Polynesians adopted the cumbersome conventions of Western dress and many of the restrictive canons of Western morality. Despite this they have still not become complete prisoners of the Guilt Cult. When writer James Michener visited the islands he was delighted to find that their attitude to sex was still characterized by a delightful lack of taboos and inhibitions. Describing his experiences in *Return to Paradise*, he reports that youngsters of either sex remained free to indulge in heterosexual activities providing they did not

207

commit incest. Any love children born of these unions were gladly adopted by older couples who had no offspring. No stigma of illegitimacy attached to these children, for the islanders had no concept of bastardy. Throughout the island the parents' attitude towards their children's sexual behaviour was one of complete acceptance; so much so, Michener reports, that 'fathers built their daughters separate cabins so they could be alone for their courting.'

This attitude of parental *laissez-faire* may be difficult for Westerners to understand. But it is fairly typical of the native approach to childhood sexuality. Many primitive societies believe that unless youngsters are allowed to experiment with sex early in their lives, they will not mature properly or be able to have children. For this reason the Chewa tribe of Africa provide their children with huts some distance from the village where, with complete parental approval, they can retire and play at being husbands and wives. These cohabitational Wendy houses are also supplied elsewhere in Africa by the Ila tribe, where it is reported that there are no virgins after the age of ten. On the Trobriand Islands youngsters are encouraged to make overt expression of their sexuality well before they reach the age of puberty, but they are allowed to marry only after they have established a compatible and affectionate relationship, and had several years of satisfactory sexual intimacy. In this way the risk of sexual pathology and marital discord is minimized.

The Marquesan people of Polynesia learn, when young, physical skills of sexual intercourse, just as they master the art of basket making, weaving, house building or hunting, by copying the example of their parents.

Harry Harlow, in his famous series of experiments on rhesus monkeys, clearly demonstrated that while sex is an instinctive primate drive, its expression is a learned pattern of behaviour, like the song call of a thrush or nightingale. Monkeys learn how to mate and how to conduct themselves in sexual encounters with the opposite sex, by copying the behaviour of their parents. If they are reared in isolation they fail to develop the appropriate sociosexual skills. Harlow found that the males he raised in cages completely segregated from the rest of the colony showed a complete lack of sexual know-how. When they were introduced to sexually mature females, some showed no amorous inclination whatsoever while others tried to mount them from the front or side. The maladroit behaviour of these animals was due entirely to their lack of practical guidance in the amatory arts. The same educational hiatus may be the root cause of much human sexual conflict and distress.

Youngsters in the Western world today are provided with an increasing amount of academic sex instruction, but are given precious little chance of gaining any practical tuition and experience, except in a purely furtive way. This is like giving a youngster a 'Teach Yourself to Swim' manual without letting him go for a dip. In this way he may not come to any great harm, but equally well he'll never learn to swim. If we want our children to avoid sexual hang-ups and develop a vigorous and healthy attitude to sex, we must allow them the chance to experiment while they're still young. When they start to masturbate we should be grateful that their sexuality is developing along normal lines, rather than be fearful lest the practice should stunt their growth or turn them into depraved libertines. And when they start to show an interest in the opposite sex, even if we don't follow the example of the Chewan people and provide them with gazebos in the garden where they can do their courting, at least we can support them in their first, exciting heterosexual love affairs. Sooner or later the tender kisses and caresses will make way for full sexual union. This we must also accept, providing they adopt a responsible attitude, for if we school youngsters to believe that the genital organs are indecent and sexual love impure, how can we expect them as adults to suddenly shed these taboos on their wedding night? It is easy to learn patterns of behaviour in childhood, but exceedingly difficult to unlearn them as adults if they prove to be inappropriate or pernicious. Such is the force of moral education that many adults never fully overcome their childhood taboos and sexual prohibitions. As adults their bodies still believe what they were trained to accept in their formative years – that nudity is indecent, the genital ogans unclean, and sexual love impure.

In a recent poll of twenty-five-year-old Britons, carried out by a London psychologist working under the auspices of the Health Education Council, only five per cent of the women and eight per cent of the men said they were satisfied wih the sex education they had received in their youth. Attempts will no doubt be made to remedy this widespread dissatisfaction by providing more formal sex education in schools, but this will not solve the underlying problem. The future generation may have a detailed knowledge of the anatomy of the human genitalia, and a profound understanding of the mating behaviour of the birds and bees, but they will still not know what it is like to form an intimate and loving relationship with a member of the opposite sex, unless they are given the opportunity to experiment. And this most parents will not be prepared to accept. Their attitude will probably remain that of the mother who, when asked if she would mind her daughter receiving sex education at school, replied, 'Not at all, providing she's not given homework.'

Mercifully the human libido is not that easily suppressed. Such is the curiosity of the young, that most children find an outlet for their developing sexual drive at an age far earlier than their parents generally realize. A recent study of British teenagers, conducted by the Institute for Social Studies in Medical Care, showed that one in five youngsters broke the law by having intercourse before they reached the age of sixteen. Many adults may be shocked to discover the extent of this sexual precocity, but as the researchers reassuringly noted in their report, 'Most teenagers have responible attitudes to sex before marriage, even if they are not traditional ones.' The same is true of students at American universities. Here surveys reveal that 47 per cent of the women and 42 per cent of the men living in co-ed dormitories are sexually active. But again there is little evidence of promiscuity, for the liaisons the undergraduates form are normally long-term love affairs rather than casual relationships.

Once the shackles of sexual taboos are broken it will be possible to enter into responsible sexual relationships without guilt or fear. Sex will then become once more a joyous celebration of human tenderness and intimacy. This is the love which does not enslave but liberates; the eroticism which does not demean but enriches; the passion which does not exhaust but revivifies. Because their sexual relationships are fuller and more satisfying, peoples' lives will become happier, freer and more vital. Likewise, because their lives are revitalized, their sexual relationships will be enhanced. Nothing has a more powerful aphrodisiac effect than the dynamogenic way of life. Spend your life sitting idly in a chair and you'll have little energy or enthusiasm for sex. Lead an exciting, vigorous life and the chances are your libido will be as indefatigable as the sea.

Tests also show that the output of sex hormones is increased under the stimulus of vigorous exercise. Research carried out at the Gavin Institute of Medical Research in Sydney, Australia, has shown that the output of testosterone, the male sex hormone, is increased when athletes take part in vigorous swimming or rowing events. Rises in blood testosterone levels are also observed when non-athletic students pedal on a static bicycle, the levels reaching a peak after about twenty minutes of energetic cycling. This biological response may help to explain the amorous behind-the-scene activities encountered at most mixed sporting clubs. Also the conduct of the two young entrants in a mixed marathon race, faithfully recorded in *The Runner's Handbook* who, after running in tandem for the first few miles, suddenly 'veered off into the fog-shrouded bushes to prove that runners, indeed, do make better lovers.' (Is this the reason why so many marathon runners fall by the wayside?) But even less strenuous forms of exercise than swimming, rowing, cycling and marathon running appear to have an aphrodisiac effect. This was discovered when Perrier, the French mineral water company, gave a questionnaire to a group of 1700 Americans and found that 28 per cent of those who took up some form of sporting exercise noted that their sex lives had been improved by their increased level of activity.

Excitement can also act as a sexual stimulant, probably by stimulating the pituitary gland to secrete more ACTH, the master stress hormone, which in turn increases the output of androgens from the testes and adrenal cortex. In an interesting field study, psychologists at the University of Columbia invited a group of male students to cross one of two bridges thrown across the Capilano River. One of these bridges was a flimsy construction of planks slung from wire cables 230 feet above the river; the other a sturdy structure built only ten feet above the water. As the students walked over the bridges they were met halfway across by a male or female interviewer who gave them a brief psychological test and a questionnaire to complete when they returned to the campus. They were also provided with the interviewer's phone number, and told that they could get in contact if they wanted any additional information about the experiment. The test revealed a fascinating sex-linked bias in the students' responses. When the men encountered a female interviewer, they were nearly 60 per cent more likely to provide sexual responses and imagery in their replies when they met her on the dangerous bridge than when their meeting was on the stable bridge. Similarly, whereas half the men phoned the girls they had met under hazardous circumstances, only one in eight did so where their contact had been met in the less stressful situation. (When the interviewer was a male there was no difference in the sexual content of the student's stories or in the number of men who sought to contact their interviewers by phone.) This suggests that sexual arousal can be promoted by strong emotions such as anxiety and fear.

Lead an exciting and energetic existence and you'll have a more dynamic love life. Allow yourself to become inactive and withdrawn and your interest in sex will wane. Tests carried out by Professor Hans Eysenck, of the London University Psychiatry Department, have shown that extroverts make love two or three times as often as introverts. Similar findings have been obtained from research carried out by American psychologist Philip Zimbardo, which has revealed that shy women are twice as likely to be virgins as women who are less reserved and introspective.

All the evidence points to the fact that dynamic living is good for sex, and sex excellent for the dynamogenic way of life. You'll find for one thing that regular participation in sex will help you lose weight and keep your body firm and trim. As film actress Ursula Andress confessed when reporters asked her how she kept her sylphlike figure, 'Loving keeps me slim.' Farmers have similarly found that they can accelerate the weight growth of heifers by fitting them with a plastic vaginal insert. These *Hei-Gro* devices suppress oestrus and minimize sexual activity, and by doing so lead to an increased weight gain of approximately 26 per cent. Metabolic studies of humans show that the average act of intercourse uses up two hundred calories. (About as much as half an hour's jogging.) Do this three times a week and you stand to lose nearly ten pounds of surplus weight a year. If the lovemaking is more energetic and frequent, the fat will melt away quicker still. And what more enjoyable way can there be to regain a youthful figure? It is surely much better to slim by feasting in the bedroom, than by fasting in the dining room.

A full and satisfying love life is also a wonderful antidote for tension. An orgasm is rather like a hearty laugh, in that it represents an explosive discharge of energy at the end of a slow period of emotional arousal and gradually mounting tension. Comedians get their effect by achieving a steady build-up of excitement and comic expectation and then, by introducing an unexpected twist or absurd allusion, suddenly releasing the tension in a peal of uninhibited laughter. The lover's art is exactly the same. Tension is engendered during a period of erotic foreplay of gradually mounting intensity, and then cataclysmically released at the moment of coital climax. In this way both laughter and love-making act to release bodily tension. Sex may be energetic but, like a day's hiking in the mountains, also deliciously relaxing. If people led richer sex lives there would be less need for tranquillizers. If they had more time for love, they would have far less time for anxiety and hate.

A common fallacy is to mistake for physical exhaustion the detumescence which comes at the end of climactic sex. This is not debility, but a state of profound and highly beneficial relaxation. Sex is not weakening, but revivifying.

According to a traditional Hindu belief man's vital energy is concentrated in his seminal fluid. The Hindu believed that it took forty drops of blood and forty days to make one drop of semen. (This must be rather hard on boars, who may copulate four times a day and release as much as half a pint of semen with each ejaculation!) To conserve this precious life force yoga teachers have recommended the practice of *brahmacharya* (celibacy), *maithuna* (coitus reservatus), or *vajroli* (drawing back the semen into the body.) Athletes are often similarly advised by their trainers to abstain from sex before an important sporting event. Even an acknowledged authority like Dr J. L. Blonstein, President of the Medical Commission of the International Amateur Boxing Association, has given credence to this myth by saying, 'Sexual abstinence is almost essential for sporting success.' But there is no evidence whatsoever to support this statement. As Professor Manfred Steinback concluded after studying the sex lives of eight hundred athletes competing in the Munich Olympic Games, 'Coaches who think they can improve their protégés' sporting achievements by banishing them from the boudoir are wasting their time.' It takes a trained athlete only one or two minutes to recover from the exertion of lovemaking. After that brief respite there is no physiological reason why they should not perform at their peak. In fact experience shows that many athletes function more effectively after a bout of energetic lovemaking. Joe Namath, the famous American quarterback, gave a performance to remember during the 1969 Super Bowl. His bedroom performance the night before was equally memorable. When recalling his activities on the eve of the big match, he said, 'I went out and grabbed this girl and brought her back to the hotel, and we had a good time the whole night. It's good for you. It loosens you up good for the game.' Dr Craig Sharp, chief medical adviser to Britain's 1972 Olympic team, has also placed on record two cases in which athletes have leapt from the bedroom on to the track and recorded their fastest ever times. One, a middle-distance runner, established a world record an hour after making love. The other, a miler, put up a personal best time of four minutes soon after giving his all in bed.

Sex is exhilarating, and no person in reasonable health needs to fear that it will sap their stamina, strain their heart or weaken their constitution. Even marathon lovemaking isn't harmful. A man studied by Professor Kinsey engaged in sex thirty times a week for thirty years and showed no signs of ill effects whatsoever. Maintain a lively interest in sex and you'll be able to enjoy its comforts and delights as long as you live. Sex researchers have proved that anyone can remain sexually active into their ninth decade providing they remain reasonably fit and have a sufficiently stimulating partner. This will enable them 'though they may be four score years above the girdle, to be scarcely thirty beneath,' as the explorer Richard Burton wrote in *The Anatomy of Melancholy*.

A healthy sexual appetite is an integral part of the dynamogenic lifestyle. People who are sexually active and content exude an attractive animal magnetism. It shows in the bloom of their skin, the confidence of their gait, the cheerfulness of their manner, the relaxation of their posture and the ease with which they establish new relationships. Friends know when you're happy in bed. People who lead vigorous sexual lives are stimulating to be with.

Wilhelm Reich, the controversial psychoanalyst who was at one time Freud's favourite disciple, believed that all psychological illness stems from libidinal repression. According to Reichean therapists, health can be obtained only by releasing the neurotic blocks which hold back the natural flow of sexual energy. In their opinion it is this primeval driving force which gives the body its superabundant powers. This may seem an extreme view, but there is no doubt, from a study of the affective lives of history's most ebullient and creative characters, that dynamism is invariably linked with vigorous sexuality. Whether one shares the political theories of Karl Marx or not, he must be accepted as one of the most influential figures of the twentieth century. A man with a prodigious propensity for work, he also had a Promethean capacity for sex. Throughout his life Marx maintained a close and loving relationship with his wife, but also found time to seduce the family maid by whom he had an illegitimate son. At the age of forty-three, while engaged on a fund-raising campaign in the Netherlands, he threw himself into a tumultuous love affair with his twenty-four-year-old cousin. A few years later his endless quest for financial backing took him to Germany where he wooed an attractive lady by regaling her with passionate love poems. As the numerous biographies about him reveal,

Marx's zeal for social reform was matched only by his passion for sex.

Albert Einstein, another of the century's most innovative personalities, also showed more than a passing interest in the opposite sex. The great physicist had a number of attractive girlfriends with whom he sometimes stayed the night according to his housekeeper, who recently published an intimate biography about her former boss. One was an attractive Austrian blonde, many years younger than Einstein's wife, whom he took on sailing expeditions. Another with whom he maintained an intimate alliance was a wealthy Berlin widow. Wisely, Einstein gave instructions that on his death all his love letters should be destroyed.

Obviously the output of these two men was not impaired by their amorous activities, which probably acted as a spur to their creativity. This was certainly true of Janacek, the great Czech composer, whose musical genius only flowered at the age of sixty-three when he fell head-over-heels in love with Kamilla Stoesslova, the attractive young wife of an antique dealer. Under the inspiration of this heady affair he produced some of his finest music, including four highly original operas, the monumental *Glagolitic Mass*, and numerous pieces of chamber and orchestral music. Hard though he worked in the latter stages of his life, Janacek's sexual drive remained undiminished, and local legend relates that he died at the age of seventy-four while chasing an attractive lady through a wood.

While most married people are probably quite happy with their sex lives, the effusive sexual drives of dynamogenic characters cannot always be satisfied within the marital relationship. But infidelity is surely not as great a moral sin as coldness, indifference and lack of caring. To preserve the institution of marriage it is natural that we should seek to curb unrestrained promiscuity, but equally unrealistic that we should expect all partners to remain totally faithful to their mates through

217

their lives. Surveys show that somewhere between 35 and 50 per cent of married people have on occasion engaged in extramarital sex. This is not a criticism of the marital state, but a commentary on human nature and the ubiquity and strength of the sexual urge. In a humane society erring partners must be treated with tolerance and understanding. The sane attitude is that of the woman who, when asked if her husband had been faithful to her replied, 'Frequently'.

There may be times when extramarital sex may help to preserve a marriage or maintain mental health. This was appreciated even by such a stern moralist as Martin Luther, who suggested that it was legitimate for a wife to take a lover if she was unsatisfied by her husband. Her proper course of action, he suggested, was to approach her partner and say, 'See, my dear husband, thou hast deceived me and my young body and endangered my honour and salvation; before God there is no honour between us. Suffer that I maintain secret marriage with thy brother or closest friend while thou remainest my husband in name. That thy property may not fall heir to strangers, willingly be deceived by me as you have unwillingly deceived me.' Hopefully compensation like this will be less necessary when a more enlightened attitude to sex prevails. Individuals who adopt the dynamogenic programme will find their sex lives enriched and will encounter little difficulty in satisfying their mates.

The following practices, which form an intrinsic part of the dynamogenic way of life, will be of particular help to readers who have sexual problems.

● *Derive maximum pleasure from your sexuality.* Sex is one of the most enriching of all human experiences. It invigorates, inspires, relaxes, and is both the gift-wrapping of heterosexual relationships and the ribbon which binds them in place. As such it merits a much higher place than it often gets in our schedule of priorities. Why give it only the fag end of your day when you're too tired for anything else? The love life of many people is impoverished not because they suffer any intrinsic psychosexual problems, but because they rate sex of secondary importance to watching television or going out to the theatre or cinema. If these outside attractions are removed for any reason, people are forced to make their own entertainment, and frequently find much greater satisfaction in bed. In 1965, there was a total shutdown of electricity in New York. This meant no electric light, no subways, no movies, no theatre. Nine months later the local hospitals recorded a 33 to 35 per cent increase in the birthrate. In 1966 the people of Venice were confined to their homes as a result of widespread flooding. Exactly nine months later the Venetian authorities announced that 45 per cent more babies than usual had been born. The following year heavy blizzards in Chicago brought traffic to a standstill and kept people marooned in their homes. Nine months later the birth rate in Chicago soared 30 to 40 per cent. But why wait for catastrophe to strike to rediscover the joys of leisurely lovemaking? If we value the benisons of sex, why can't we voluntarily switch off the TV, pull down the blinds, slip the latch on the door and for an evening put up the no-callers sign? Then lovers will have time once more to linger and luxuriate in each other's arms.

Too much contemporary sex is hurried. Perhaps in a world of jet travel, fast food, condensed books and instamatic photographs it's inevitable that lovemaking should be conducted at the same breathless pace. An article in the Russian health magazine *Zdorovye* recommends that intercourse should last only two minutes. This may be fine if your object is simply to perpetuate the race in the briefest possible time before rushing back to continue work on the factory production line, but not if you want to enjoy a meaningful heterosexual relationship. There should never be a time limit on sex. The moment of orgasmic climax may be uncharitably brief, but the period of preliminary foreplay and post-copulatory dalliance is limitless. We should be prepared to spend eternity in our lovers' arms, like snakes which sometimes remain locked in a copulatory embrace for anything up to twenty-two hours. The early love manuals assumed that disciples of the amatory arts would spend time to develop their skills. The *Kama Sutra* devotes pages to the early stages of sexual congress, when without any sense of haste lovers exchange long lingering kisses on the lips, forehead, eyes, cheeks, throat, bosom and chest. This theme was upheld by gynaecologist Dr H. Van de Velde, whose famous 1930s textbook *Ideal Marriage* did so much to shape our parents' view of sex. He too stressed the importance of pre-copulatory arousal and described in some detail the lover's kiss when a couple 'sometimes for hours mutually explore and caress the inside of each other's mouths with their tongues as profoundly as possible.'

Young people may still find time to share these erotic delights, but what about people past the first flush of youth? For many, lovemaking today is pared down to its final climactic moment – a brief reflex spasm of the muscles. Shorn in this way of all its tenderness and warmth the sexual exchange becomes as meaningless as a shaggy dog story with its initial preamble censored and only its punchline intact. Women suffer particularly from this unromantic, mechanistic approach to sex. Their most frequent complaint to doctors and agony columnists nowadays is not that they get too little sex, but that their partners provide them with too little tenderness and affection. Many men, in their constant preoccupation with work, spend more time shaving than they do making love to their wives. If this is their scale of values they may make a fortune, but they also stand the risk of ending up frustrated, clean-shaven cuck-olds.

● *Take delight in your body*. Sex is distasteful for some people because it involves an animalistic coupling of two sweating, writhing bodies. How can it be an act of beauty when it entails the exposure of naked flesh and such close involvement with the organs of excretion? How can a nicely brought up person relax and enjoy such a bestial pastime, except as a conjugal duty, or a means of begetting children? Anyone who holds such repressive ideas, or clings to childhood taboos against touching or even exposing the genital organs, is obviously going to be disadvantaged when he or she attempts to form an adult sexual relation-ship. Delight in sex involves delight in the human body and a complete acceptance of all its various parts. Nothing about the human frame is, or ever could be, indecent.

We are trained in childhood to place strict limits on our physical contact with other people, and to maintain a complete bar on any exposure or handling of the genital organs. So strong is this early discipline that many adults still find nude bathing embarras-sing, masturbation wicked, and sexual intercourse distasteful. These unhealthy interdictions need to be banished before a full and satisfactory sex life can be enjoyed. Many people have been enabled to do this by joining encounter groups. These have provided the permissive arenas in which people have been able to bare their bodies in public and overcome their taboos against touching and being touched. More specific therapy has been provided by sex therapists such as Betty Dodson of New York. She has formed small groups of women and painstakingly trained them to overcome their sexual hang-ups. As a result, most of the previously non-orgasmic women who attend the sessions are helped to reach a climax by self-stimulation. Having achieved this, they invariably find it easier to obtain fulfilment in their normal heterosexual relationships.

But it would be a grave mistake to think of sex as a purely genital act. In fact many contemporary sexual relationships are impoverished not through excessive prudery, but because they involve the short-lived coupling of two sexual organs, rather than the timeless mingling of two bodies, minds and souls. True eroticism is not limited to the skilful manipulation of the penis and clitoris, but embraces also the exchange of loving looks, gentle words and tender caresses. Sexuality is a total body response, which brings into play every one of the five senses. Few men realize the value of softly spoken words of endearment, which can bring some women to a climax without any form of stimulation. The sense of smell is another much neglected sensory stimulant, particularly now it has become customary to obliterate all the natural body odours with perfumed talcs, antiperspirants and deodorants. Historians tell that King Henry III of France was first attracted to Marie de Clèves by her delightful body odour. He was attending the wedding feast of the King of Navarre and Marguerite de Valois, and at one point in the festivities retired to a side chamber to get a brief respite after a particularly energetic spell of dancing. To mop his brow he picked up a garment which had been discarded only a few minutes before by an equally limp Marie de Clèves. Still wet with her sweat, the garment had such a heady aroma that the king experienced an immediate and passionate attraction for its owner.

Unless we make full use of our senses, life is stripped of its richness, colour and variety. So too is sex. And one of the finest ways of enhancing the sexual act is to enjoy to the full the sight, touch, smell and sound of the one you love.

● *Let yourself go and give vent to your feelings.* When you're making love, it's better to let your hair down and do what comes naturally than to follow the well-meaning but stilted instructions of sex therapists. Never be a mean and measured lover. If you want to fix your partner's buttocks in a vice-like grip, don't be deterred from doing so because the procedure isn't mentioned in your favourite manual of sex technique. If your mate doesn't like it he or she will soon let you know. In sex there's a time for tenderness and equally well a time for passion, and only you are likely to know the appropriate moment for expressing either emotion. A degree of aggression can be observed in the copulatory behaviour of most mammals, and far from being inimical to the sex act, this generally acts as a powerful amoratory stimulant. Stallions often nip the withers of brood mares before they prepare to mount, sea-lions bite each other's necks and male sheep clench their teeth firmly in the fleece and skin of their chosen ewe. In some mammals coitus only takes place after a prolonged chase and painful struggle. When a male mink wants to express his amorous intent, he sinks his teeth clean through the pelt of his inamorata. Not surprisingly her initial reaction is a vigorous attempt to escape. But generally after a protracted battle the more powerful male overcomes her struggles and achieves penetration. Encounters like these give the sex war a more literal meaning, and make our own traditional romp around the bedroom and playful smack on the behind seem as gentle and refined as a Sunday School outing. A little rough and tumble, nipping, struggling and slapping can add spice to the sex act, and becomes pathological only when it causes lasting damage or is unacceptable to either partner. Boisterous behaviour like this may not win friends or influence people in everyday life, but it can work wonders in the bedroom.

When consenting adults make love they should cease to be selfconscious, and should temporarily abandon all the restraints of normal civilized society. If in the moment of ultimate passion you want to grunt or groan like a contented sow, do so. Don't worry about what the neighbours might think. It's your partner's reactions that count, and they're likely to find your ecstatic moans the ultimate turn-on, and a delightful compliment to their own sexual prowess. Be bold enough too to act out some of your hidden fantasies. If you dream of making love in a hayrick, in the shower, or with your body smothered in ice-cream and chocolate sauce, why hold back? In the field of sexual activity a little of what you fancy will almost certainly do you good.

Some people are physically too rigid and restrained to act in this liberated way. As Wilhelm Reich revealed, they protect themselves by holding themselves in a straightjacket of muscular tension. They erect a 'body armouring' which prevents them from feeling pain, but also stops them from experiencing pleasure. By contracting their diaphragm they hold back the tears, and by tensing their pelvic and abdominal muscles they still the rumbles of fear, and the sinking feelings of rejection. But by maintaining tension in these muscles they prevent themselves from experiencing total orgasmic satisfaction. Relief in such cases can only be obtained by unlocking the restraining muscular tensions. This can be done by performing deep breathing exercises (see page 266) and by unshackling the pelvic musculature. Reichean therapists offer a number of techniques designed to make the pelvis come more fully alive. But the same effect can be obtained far more simply by indulging in bouts of unrestrained laughter. (If you find this difficult to do in the cold light of day, go into a shower and laugh continuously and uproariously until the tears flow down your cheeks.) Belly dancing is another excellent way of mobilizing the pelvis. So too is hula hula dancing, the jive and most Latin American dance forms. When the ladies of the Egyptian harems peformed their sinuous belly dances they not only stimulated their masters' ardours, but also freed the tensions in their own bodies, so that they could more fully enjoy love-making. Perform these liberating exercises and you'll help to make bad sex good, and good sex better.

● *Live a varied life.* Monotonous routine is the death of many sexual unions. This at least is the verdict of sex researchers Masters and Johnson, who claim that boredom is 'probably the most constant factor in the loss of the ageing male's interest in sexual perform-ance with his partner.' This may explain the ancient practice of placing impotent elderly men in the company of lively young maidens. The belief at the time was that inhaling the young girl's breath helped to restore the old men's lost virility, but it seems far more likely that their potency was recaptured by the youngster's freshness and charm. The cure was tried on the ailing King David, but unfortunately he was too far gone to appreciate the stimulus of being placed side by side in bed with the young virgin Abishag. No doubt he inhaled her breath before he died, but because of his debilitated state he 'knew her not', and was therefore unable to derive full benefit from the experiment. The experience of L. Claudius Hermip was much more satisfactory. According to the inscription of an ancient tomb-stone, Hermip 'lived one hundred and fifteen years with the aid of the breath of young women, to the surprise of physicians.' On the strength of this remarkable achievement the engraver advised all who read the gravestone to 'Lead your life accordingly.'

Variety is one of the main pathways to sexual excitement and a key principal of dynamogenic living. Even lobster thermidor would get boring if you had it for each and every meal. So does sex if it's always taken in the same manner, place and time. Psychiatrists have found that they can cure deviants of their sexual perversions by subjecting them to a massive overdose of their favoured fetishes. Two American psychologists, W. L. Marshall and K. Lippens, cured a rapist of his uncontrollable passion for women in nylon stockings by subjecting him to an undiluted diet of nylon stockings. For hours on end he was permitted to do nothing but masturbate or fantasize while thinking of gossamer-stockinged legs. After six sessions he claimed that he was cured and 'could not bear to go through that boring procedure again.' For safety's sake he was subjected to a further three treatments, at which point he was 'no longer sexually excited by seeing women wearing stockings or panti-hose.' The response to sensory stimulation follows the law of diminishing returns. Repeat a sensation often enough in unchanging form and it will quickly cease to have a stimulating effect. Get out of bed and put on your clothes and a few minutes later you'll cease to notice that you're dressed. Go through the same sexual routine, lights-out-in-bed-at-eleven-o'clock-on-a-Sunday-night-in-the-missionary-position, and you'll soon begin to wish that you were back downstairs watching the television.

To retain its freshness, gourmet sex must be as varied as the diet in a five-star restaurant. If you feel amorous at times and in places where you would not normally make love, why not give vent to your feelings? Anything rather than submit to the stultifying boredom of routine, which kills passion and slowly strangles life itself. We have at our command a greater range of sexual techniques and copulatory positions than any other animal. Using them to the full will greatly enrich our love lives, for as King Louis XV's physician rightly said, 'Change is the greatest aphrodisiac of all.'

11

High-Vite or Low-Vite?

By now you should have a fairly clear idea of the sort of life you lead. Either you're a High-Vite, leading a dynamogenic way of life, or you're a Low-Vite, following an existence which is largely sedentary and hypokinetic. This is a fundamental differentiation which determines both your current physical and mental well-being, and also your future health status. If you're a High-Vite you're likely to be lively, slim and happy, with an above-average chance of leading a long and successful life. If you're a Low-Vite you're prone to tiredness, obesity, heart disease, rheumatic aches and pains and premature ageing. Fortunately these classifications are not irrevocably fixed. It's possible to adopt the dynamogenic programme at any time of life, and so join the small, privileged band of High-Vites, who possibly make up no more than five per cent of the adult population of the Western world.

But before elaborating the dynamogenic plan in detail, determine your present vitality rating by completing the following questionnaire. (Record your responses on a sheet of paper, giving a 'Yes' or 'No' answer to each question.)

Dynamogenic questionnaire
1 Do you walk more than two hours a week?
2 Do you normally go to bed when you are tired and wake fully refreshed?
3 Can you bend down and touch your toes?
4 Have you made any radical changes in your hairstyle or dress in the last five years?
5 Do you find it easy to let your hair down and laugh,

shout and generally play around?

6 Are you a non-smoker?

7 Have you an all-absorbing interest in music, stamp collecting, vintage cars, antiquarian books, pottery or other similar subject?

8 Are you fond of sweets, ice cream, biscuits and cake?

9 Do you long for more time to accomplish all you want to achieve?

10 Do you frequently climb the stairs rather than use the escalator?

11 Do you get up in the morning feeling fit rather than aching and stiff?

12 When you go to the doctor are you most satisfied when you come away without a prescription for drugs?

13 Have you taken up a new hobby or sport in the last three years?

14 Would you willingly take part in a fancy dress competition?

15 Are you currently living without the aid of sleeping pills, tranquillizers and anti-depressants?

16 Do you spend as much time as possible out of doors?

17 Do you sometimes vary the route you take to the office or shops, and read a different daily paper?

18 Can you grip your hands behind your back, left hand passing behind your left ear, right arm passing behind your back?

19 Do you take part at least twice a week in an active sport such as cycling, swimming, jogging or tennis?

20 Do you make friends easily?

21 Are you sometimes so totally absorbed in what you are doing that you lose all sense of time?

22 Do you have a daily ration of either fresh fruit or salad?

23 Do you, as far as possible, avoid using labour-saving gadgets such as automatic dishwashers, electric toothbrushes and remote control TV channel selectors?

24 When you wake up in the morning do you normally

look forward to the challenges that the day may bring?

25 Do you drink in moderation (less than two pints of beer a day, or half a bottle of wine or three and a half measures of spirits)?

26 Can you sit for two hours in a car seat or easy chair without suffering backache?

27 Have you more than three intimate friends?

28 Do you live in the present rather than wishing you could return to the good old days?

29 Are you engaged at present in studying a new subject, or learning a new skill?

30 When you're in pain do you always try to remedy the underlying cause of your discomfort before you resort to taking pain-killing drugs?

31 Can you squat down on your haunches with knees fully flexed and heels resting on the ground?

32 Have you in the last week exercised hard enough to get out of breath?

33 Do you sometimes cry over a film, book or piece of music?

34 Do you sometimes make love in the middle of the day in a location other than the bedroom?

35 Have you during the last year had a dip in a cold pool, or taken a cold shower or bath?

Scoring (Score one point for every 'Yes', no points for a 'No'.)

Points total		How you rate
1–5	Extremely low	The life you lead at present is unhealthily inactive, monotonous and dull.
6–10	Low	Your physical and mental well-being is suffering considerably from your hypokinetic lifestyle.

11–15	Below average	You follow a conventional sedentary existence and would benefit greatly by adopting a more dynamic approach to life.
16–20	Average	You have escaped the worst pitfalls of hypokinetic living, but would still derive marked gains in health and happiness by pursuing a more dynamic lifestyle.
21–25	Above average	Your life is more vigorous than most people's, but you are liable to suffer occasionally from the effects of sedentary living and should try to increase your vitality rating.
26–30	High	Your life is lively and stimulating, but could be enhanced by the injection of a little more vitality, novelty and excitement.
31–35	Exceptionally high	You lead a life which is remarkably energetic, varied and exciting.

By completing the above questionnaire you will have a rough estimation of your vitality rating, and can see how far your current way of life departs from the dynamogenic ideal. (After following the dynamogenic programme for a year, repeat the test to see how much your scores have improved.) A study of your responses to the questions will also reveal certain of your characteristic personality traits, and highlight those areas of your life that are in most urgent need of revision. To extract this vital information and get a clearer picture of your individual personality profile, carry out the following analysis:

Behavioural profile

Characteristic Scoring (Add the scores from these questions, allotting 1 point for 'Yes', no points for 'No')

Characteristic	Scoring	
Active/idle	1,10,19,23,32	Scores of three or under reveal an excessively inactive life. Stress dynamogenic step one (page 235).
Emotionally extroverted/reserved	5,14,20,27,33	Scores of three or under reveal a reserved personality; follow advice contained in dynamogenic step four (page 257).
Supple/stiff	3,11,18,26,31	Scores of three or under show that you are excessively stiff. Follow dynamogenic step six (page 269).
Natural/artificial	2,8,16,22,35	Scores of three or under expose the artificiality of your current lifestyle. Place particular emphasis on dynamogenic step two (page 239).
Varied/routine	4,13,17,28,34	Scores of three or under reveal an element of monotony in your life. Follow dynamogenic step four (page 257).

Biologically self-sufficient/ drug-dependent	6,12,15,25,30	Scores of three or under suggest that you have become excessively dependent on drugs. Place particular emphasis on dynamogenic step three (page 252).
Lively/dull	7,9,21,24,29	Scores of three or under reveal that there is too little enthusiasm and passion in your life. Stress dynamogenic step four (page 257).

Having determined your personality profile, and estimated your vitality rating, it is now time to describe in detail the seven basic steps of dynamogenic living.

12

The Seven Steps to Dynamogenic Living

By now the principles and precepts of dynamogenic living should be patently clear. To enjoy the benefits of this vigorous and healthy mode of life, it's not necessary to count calories, shun fatty foods, swallow vitamin pills, or carry out an endless examination of the inner workings of your psyche. All that's required is the acquisition of the habit of vital living.

During the preceding chapters a total of thirty-one separate measures have been suggested for overcoming the most common banes of hypokinetic living – tiredness, depression, anxiety, rheumatism, obesity, heart disease, lack of success, premature ageing and sexual dysfunction. Although they can be considered in isolation, each of these precepts forms an integral part of the dynamogenic way of life. Anyone incorporating these principles into his or her daily pattern of living will be well on the way to achieving greater health, happiness and success.

At this stage a clearer, more precise, blueprint is obviously needed, and in the pages which follow the principles of dynamogenic living are encapsulated in seven basic steps. These embrace all the precepts outlined in the previous chapters together with several additional measures which are considered necessary to compensate for the inactivity of most contemporary life.

Establish these seven simple habits as part of your automatic daily routine and your life will be completely revitalized.

Dynamogenic step one: Take a minimum of ten activity units a week

To overcome the maladies of modern life it's necessary to keep active. This isn't just a question of joining a tennis club or taking up jogging, but of making a far more fundamental change in lifestyle. In the past manufacturers have considered it a virtue to flood the market with labour-saving gadgets. Now this trend must be reversed. The requisites of health demand that we should reintroduce more physical effort into our daily lives.

There are innumerable ways in which this can be done. Stand up rather than sit down when you answer the telephone. Park the car a few hundred yards from your final destination and travel the rest of the journey by foot. Sit in a rocking chair at night instead of a fixed fireside chair. This will help you lose weight (see page 131) and also improve your circulation. Varicose veins are one of the curses of sedentary living. The veins in the legs are equipped with unidirectional valves. These allow the blood to be driven up towards the heart whenever the calves contract, but prevent it from flowing back again towards the feet. This ensures that every time the calves contract deoxygenated blood is drained from the legs and driven back to the heart. Tests show that when a tracer dye is injected into the veins around the ankle it shows little tendency to move so long as the legs remain inert. But within seconds of the leg muscles being brought into active use the dye can be detected coursing through the veins of the groin. Television has been justly blamed for causing an increase in varicose veins and thrombosis, because the leg muscles are scarely used while sitting. Use a rocking chair and this hazard is greatly reduced. If you're a sufferer from backache, you'll also find that rocking helps to ease your spinal aches and pains (see page 107).

The great attraction of all dynamogenic cures is that they're safe, simple, cheap and multipotent. If you take a laxative, it may loosen your bowels but you can't expect it to relieve your insomnia or cure your headaches. But if you step up your level of physical exercise by whatever means you choose, your health will improve in every possible respect. You may take up jogging simply to safeguard the health of your heart, but in doing so you will inevitably develop a trimmer figure and feel less tense, more energetic and generally fitter. In the same way, the rocking chair you buy may be designed primarily to ease the pain in your back, but in using it you'll also improve your circulation, soothe away your bodily tensions and shed a few pounds of surplus flesh. Maybe you go ballroom dancing basically as a way of improving your figure or enlarging your social circle. But whatever the original motivation, the beneficial effects of dancing will not be restricted to these initial goals. If regularly performed it will add considerably to your physical and mental well-being, and make you more lively. It will also increase your spontaneity, give you a chance to express your fantasies and feelings in a culturally acceptable way, and improve your social poise and skills in communicating with others by non-verbal means.

Providing you lead a suitably active life it doesn't matter whether you choose to dance, swim, climb mountains, hike, aqualung, ski, ride a bicycle or sail an ocean-going yacht. Choose whatever sport you like, and as long as it gives your body the level of exercise it needs so badly, all the benefits of dynamogenic living will be yours.

If you're a lumberjack or coal miner it's just possible that your daily labours provide you with sufficient exercise to keep you in perfect shape. But if you're a teacher, architect, clerk, factory worker, housewife, shop assistant or any other of the hundreds of other largely sedentary occupations, the chances are that your work is insufficiently energetic to maintain your body in perfect health. In this case you must compensate by injecting more vigorous activity into your leisure hours. Possibly

ACTIVITY	TIME (IN MINUTES) TO RECORD ONE ACTIVITY UNIT
Badminton	35
Basketball	20
Canoeing (Slow)	66*
(Fast)	28
Climbing	15
Cycling (Gentle)	40
(Vigorous)	25
Dancing (Slow)	40
(Lively)	30
Gardening (Gentle weeding)	45
(Digging)	30
Golf	50*
Gymnastics (Gentle keep–fit)	30
(Vigorous exercise)	20
Hiking	30
Horse riding (Walking)	80*
(Trotting)	24
(Galloping)	20
Rowing (50 strokes a minute)	30
(95 strokes a minute)	20
(Peak effort)	10
Running (Jogging)	30
(Fast cross country)	20
Sawing wood	24
Skating (Gentle)	30
(Fast)	20
Skiing	26
Squash	25
Swimming (Leisurely)	30
(Fast)	20
Table tennis	40
Ten pin bowling	56*
Tennis (Singles)	26
(Doubles)	34
Walking (Gentle)	50*
(Brisk)	30
Wrestling	14

*Activities marked with an asterisk are unlikely to be sufficiently strenuous to exert a training effect on the heart.

you could keep yourself relaxed by the occasional round of golf, and could stop yourself putting on weight by taking a gentle hour's stroll each day, but you've got to exercise more vigorously than this if you want to keep your heart and lungs in peak working order. Tests show that to ensure cardiorespiratory fitness the average sedentary person needs to expend an extra two thousand calories a week in brisk physical activity. The simplest way of monitoring this output is to use the table on page 237, which shows the average number of calories used in a wide range of activities. For convenience the energy expenditure is measured in Activity Units (AUs), each of which represents an outlay of two hundred calories. With this simple method of calculation all that's necessary is to ensure that you exercise enough each week to amass a total of ten AUs. (To begin with you may find it useful to keep a daily record of the number of AUs you score, but eventually this will become unnecessary as you grow accustomed to maintaining the necessary level of physical activity.)

If you're sadly out of condition at present – overweight, with raised blood pressure and a heavy consumer of cigarettes – make sure you follow the advice given in pages 159–61 and get yourself in better shape before you embark upon your cardiorespiratory conditioning programme. Take care too that you don't overdo things in the first few weeks of training. You'll greatly reduce the risk of injury and strain by following the progressive plan of exercise outlined in the chart opposite.

Once you've built up to ten AUs a week, this must be maintained every week of your life, come rain or shine. If it's too wet to play tennis, go for an indoor swim instead. If you're away on business and can't find a suitable squash partner, pull on a tracksuit and jog around the nearest park. If blisters prevent you from rowing, go for a spin on a bike. And if your partner complains that sport is taking up too much of your time, settle for an evening's dancing together instead.

Age at start of programme	Weeks													
	1	2	3	4	5	6	7	8	9	10	11	12	13	14
Under 30	4	4	5	6	8	10								
30–40	4	4	5	5	6	7	8	10						
40–50*	2	3	3	4	5	6	7	8	9	10				
50–60*	1	2	2	3	4	5	6	7	8	9	10			
60–70*	1	1	2	2	3	4	5	6	7	8	9	10		
Over 70*	1	1	2	2	2	3	3	4	5	6	7	8	9	10

*At these ages the programme should be temporarily discontinued, and medical advice sought, if the exercise taken gives rise to chest pain, respiratory distress, palpitations or feelings of faintness.

If sickness prevents you from getting your full allowance of exercise, revert to a gentler training schedule and slowly build up to your standard allotment of ten AUs a week. If you're out of action for a month, for example, drop back four weeks on the exercise chart and then gradually work back to your full programme by following the increments of exercise suggested as being suitable for your age group.

Dynamogenic step two: Lead a more natural life
Machines have revolutionized our world. In some ways the technological advances of the last two centuries have greatly enriched our lives, but in other respects they have left us much the poorer. We have now grown so dependent on our mechanical toys that we find it exceedingly difficult to exist without them. When an acute shortage of petrol hit the west coast of America, the incidence of suicide in California soared. People felt impotent without their cars – a condition doctors quickly

labelled the 'gasoline neurosis syndrome.' Similarly, when a team of West German research workers assembled a group of 184 volunteers and challenged them to stop watching television for a year they were amazed to discover the extent of dependence on TV. Most found the craving so overpowering that they had to break their self-imposed abstinence after only a few weeks, and none could survive for more than six months without their favourite anodyne. Now there is no doubt that television and the motor car are two of the greatest fruits of twentieth-century technology, but they should not be allowed to monopolize our lives or endanger our health.

People claim that their lives are so rushed nowadays that they're forced to travel everywhere by car, but tests reveal that in most cities the bicycle is a much speedier form of transport than the car. Surveys carried out by the Consumers' Association show that cyclists moved through the London rush hour traffic at an average speed of 14 km/h (9 mph), which is considerably faster than the 4 km/h (2½ mph) logged by users of public transport. Get yourself a bike and you'll travel quicker around the cities, and also lose your dependence on petrol shortages and road hold-ups. In addition you'll save money, cause less pollution of the atmosphere, improve your health and lose weight. (Ex-racing cyclist Chris Harvey lost 4·5 kilos (10 lbs) in a single week, and took 76 mm (3 in) off his 110-cm (44-in) waist, by pedalling furiously around Hyde Park in his lunch hour.)

Spending less time watching television is also likely to improve your general health, because the hours you spend away from the box will almost certainly be devoted to more active tasks. (Apart from sleeping, it's difficult to envisage *any* recreational occupation more passive than watching television!) A short while ago the *Daily Mail* carried out the fascinating experiment of offering four families a prize of £200 if they could stop watching TV for an entire month. All succeeded in winning the bribe, and after they'd overcome their initial withdrawal symptoms settled down to a recreational lifestyle which was noticeably more creative, active and relaxed. Ron Cooper, a forty-year-old bakery area sales manager, spent his spare time decorating his lounge, which had been waiting to be painted for nearly a year. Keeping busy in this way reduced his smoking by half. Meantime his eleven-year-old son Paul busied himself skateboarding, and spent so much more time at the local adventure playground that he was elected to its managing committee. And younger daughters Mandy and Julie, instead of arguing over which TV programme to watch, played together as they'd never done before, and became much better friends as a result. Teachers also commented on the marked improvement in the children's homework during the weeks when they were without TV. Similar changes were noticed in the Hurst household. Without TV to distract him, Ray Hurst, a thirty-two-year-old civil servant, got down at last to writing a children's play, while Bernice, his wife, collected and tested cheesecake recipes for a book she'd always intended to compile. And their children, no longer mesmerized by the electronic eye, played in a way which was noticeably more lively, creative – and noisy! During his month of TV deprivation John Summerskill, a thirty-nine-year-old toolmaker, took up amateur dramatics, while Gudrun, his thirty-five-year-old wife, joined a yoga class and started writing humorous magazine articles. They noticed how much more boisterous their six-year-old son became once he was released from the soporific grip of the flickering screen.

People who lessen their dependence on cars, TV and other mechanical devices inevitably lead more active lives. They also make greater use of their legs. Regular walking was advocated in Chapter 3 as a tonic for depression, and in Chapter 6 as a means of weight reduction. (If you walk briskly for half an hour every day you'll burn up approximately 1,400 calories a week, which is equivalent to a weight loss of nearly twenty-two pounds a year.) Vigorous walking also has a beneficial effect on the heart. When carried out regularly it strengthens the cardiac muscle and improves the coronary circulation. This was clearly demonstrated when London doctors took electrocardiograms (ECGs) of nearly nine thousand male civil servants aged between forty and sixty-four. Examination of these tracings revealed that people were far less likely to have abnormal ECGs if they walked regularly to and from work. Among the people who walked for more than twenty minutes a day the incidence of ECG irregularities was only four per cent but the proportion rose to five per cent in those whose walking was limited to under ten minutes a day, and to six per cent in those who got no walking at all. Rediscover your legs and you'll be slimmer, more relaxed and less likely to suffer coronary disease.

The reversion to a more natural existence means more than dispensing with unnecessary pieces of mechanical equipment, like escalators, automatic car washes and electric shoe polishers. It also involves establishing a closer rapport with Nature. Few people realize how enervating the atmosphere can be within a modern centrally heated home or office. The air around us is normally teeming with electrically charged particles or ions, which are produced as a result of storms, the bombardment of cosmic rays, the steady release of radioactive substances in the soil, ultraviolet radiation from the sun, and the constant frictional movement of water, wind and sand. Every time we breathe we draw these ions into our lungs, from where they pass into the bloodstream and are transported throughout the body. Their effect is to stimulate metabolism and facilitate the activity of many of the body's most essential enzyme systems. The exact effect an ion has depends upon the charge it carries. Ions bearing negative charges increase the oxygenation of the blood and provide the sort of lift you'd expect to get from inhaling a whiff of pure oxygen. Those carrying positive charges have the reverse effect, decreasing the tissue uptake of oxygen and tending to make people feel tired, stuffy, irritable and depressed. Fortunately the atmosphere normally contains a preponderance of negative ions, but the ratio of positive ions can build up before a storm, or when a hot, dry wind is blowing such as the French *mistral* or the Egyptian *khamsin*. This leads to feelings of headache, irritability and pronounced lethargy. The same depressing conditions often prevail in centrally heated rooms, because ion depletion arises as a result of the introduction of metal ducts and fans in heating systems, and the use of synthetic furnishing fabrics which generate static electricity. This means that many people are spending a large part of their lives in an artificially debilitating environment. As Dr Albert Kreuger, Professor of Bacteriology at the University of California has said, 'People travelling to work in polluted air, spending hours a day in offices and factories, and living their leisure hours in urban dwellings, inescapably breathe ion-depleted air for substantial portions of their lives. There is increasing evidence that this ion depletion leads to discomfort, enervation and lassitude, and loss of mental and physical efficiency.'

The answer to this dilemma is to spend as much time as possible in the open air and, whenever possible, to throw open wide the windows and doors of houses, shops, offices and factories. Some people may complain that this will cause an unhealthy draught, and make them catch a cold or chill, but there is no substance whatsoever in these old-fashioned ideas. Tests conducted at the Medical Research Council's Common Cold Research Unit, Salisbury, have shown that the likelihood of volunteers contracting an artificially induced cold are not increased by wearing damp socks, sitting about in rain-soaked clothing, or taking a hot bath and then lingering for half an hour in a chilly corridor clad only in a dripping wet bathing costume. In fact it seems probable that infections with the common cold virus are more likely to arise in centrally heated rooms than in environments that are cold and damp. A cheese factory in Wales has observed that employees working in the dry, hot atmosphere of their offices have twice as many colds a year as those working in the work's cold storage rooms. And army authorities have discovered that the sickness rate of regiments billetted under canvas often mounts the moment they're transferred to centrally heated barrack blocks.

In many ways we would be better off if we turned our central heating systems down and kept our bodies a little cooler. For one thing we would almost certainly work more effectively. In experiments at the University of Cincinnati by Professor Clarence Mills, the behaviour of rats brought up in a cool environment was compared with that of rats reared in conditions of tropical heat. These tests revealed that the animals who were allowed to keep their cool were more active, matured more quickly, began their sexual cycles sooner, were more resistant to infection, and quicker to solve maze puzzles. Exposure to cold is also a stimulus to human activity, partly because it increases the uptake of oxygen in the lungs, and partly because it provokes the thyroid and adrenal glands to increase their production of two of the body's most powerful natural stimulants, thyroxine and adrenaline. Heat, on the other hand, tends to have a soporific effect. Tests on a group of twenty-seven healthy babies showed that they sucked less vigorously at the breast when the temperature in their immediate environment rose from 26°C (80°F) to 32°C (90°F). Paediatricians have likewise noted that infants are significantly less active when they are heavily clothed than when their unclad bodies are left exposed to the air.

Nudity is stimulating and delightfully sensuous, as Professor J. C. Flugel, the eminent psychoanalyst, discovered when he conducted an enquiry of people's responses to going about as Nature intended. When they exposed their bodies to the gentle play of sun, wind and air, they described the sensation as 'glowing', 'heavenly', 'perfectly delightful' and 'like breathing in happiness'. Shedding your clothes as frequently as possible will also expose your body to the sun's health-giving ultra-violet rays. This acts as a multipurpose tonic. In the first place sunlight is the cheapest, simplest and most natural of all bactericidal agents. Taken in regular doses it will rid the skin of many of the germs responsible for causing pimples, boils and acne spots. It also helps to remedy psoriasis, one of the most disfiguring of chronic skin complaints, a team of doctors from Copenhagen having reported that 93 per cent of psoriatic Danes lost their unsightly skin lesions after spending a sunshine holiday by the Dead Sea. The powerful germ-killing action of sunlight also reduces the incidence of respiratory infection. This has been confirmed by tests which show that schoolchildren suffer fewer coughs and colds when their classrooms are irradiated with ultraviolet light.

Another important function of sunlight is the creation within the skin of Vitamin D. This vital food factor is essential for the formation of healthy bones, and is created in significant quantities when ultraviolet light irradiates the skin and reacts with a fatty substance called ergosterol, which is always present in the deeper layers of the skin. This explains why the disease of rickets is so common in children living in sun-starved cities, and why so many housebound elderly people develop osteomalacia, a condition characterized by a painful softening of the bones. At one time it was believed that this disorder was due solely to a dietary deficiency of Vitamin D, but recent studies carried out by the Medical Research Council have emphasized the important role played by sunlight deprivation. These investigations have shown that whereas many people of pensionable age exist on diets deficient in Vitamin D, only those who are starved of sunlight develop clinical signs of osteomalacia. This deficiency also predisposes to fractures. In recent years there has been a twelve per cent increase in broken legs among British senior citizens, an increase which a team of doctors in Bristol attribute in large measure to the accumulation of ozone in the stratosphere, which filters off many of the sun's ultraviolet rays before they have a chance of reaching the earth.

There's also a strong possibility that exposure to sunlight acts as a spur to sexual activity. Biologists have noted that the level of male sex hormones in stickleback fish increases on exposure to light, and that the testes of the highly fecund hamster shrink to about a quarter of their normal size when they're kept in darkness. They've also noted that birds which normally breed only in the spring can be made to produce a second clutch of eggs if they're irradiated with ultraviolet light during the winter. But is there any evidence that sunlight provides a stimulus for human sexual behaviour? The only confirmation of this comes from statistical studies, which show that conceptions are more likely to occur during the summer than during the sunless winter months. Thus, when public health authorities in New York analysed a series of well over a million births, they found a higher than average number of conceptions at the end of the summer, with fewest babies conceived during the spring, at the end of the dark days of winter. Maybe in view of this we should amend Tennysons's oft-quoted lines and make the summer rather than the spring the time when 'a young man's fancy lightly turns to thoughts of love'.

Sunshine is also a general metabolic stimulus, boosting the number of white blood cells in the circulation and producing a sense of exhilaration which one doctor has described as the 'I-don't-know-what's-wrong-with-me-I-feel-so-grand' feeling. And this tonic effect can be enjoyed on overcast days as well as when the skies are blue and the sun is visibly shining, for even fog and fairly dense clouds let through 20 to 50 per cent of the sun's rays. But this is not true of windows and walls, which effectively block out all the sun's ultraviolet rays. Stay indoors and you'll become as sickly as an etiolated house plant. There's an old English proverb which says, 'The sun is the finest physician, but the most difficult to make an appointment with.' To this wry statement might be added the important rider that Dr Sol never makes house calls. To derive the full benefit of the stimulus of sun, wind and air we should spend as much time as possible out of doors, dressed in as few clothes as comfort and the climate permit.

Turning down the thermostatic controls of central heating systems to 18°C (65°F) would provide another valuable metabolic stimulus, and would at the same time make a major contribution to the conservation of the world's limited store of fossil fuels. It would also help to overcome the problem of obesity, for when the environmental temperature falls we automatically stoke up our own internal fires, and increase the rate at which we burn up surplus fat. Research carried out at Bispebjerg Hospital, Copenhagen, has shown that the metabolism of lean people soars 33⅓ per cent when they're exposed to a temperature of 3°C (39°F). (Unfortunately the metabolism of fat people rises by only 2½ per cent because of their extra layer of fatty insulation.) This means that you can lose weight even when you're sitting down, providing you're sitting in a sufficiently cold environment.

A cold bath or shower is an even more powerful stimulant, increasing the rate of metabolism by as much as 80 per cent. This is an excellent way to start the day, not just because it helps to blow away the early morning cobwebs and get the metabolic fires burning, but because it also provides an excellent tonic for the circulation. However, middle-aged or elderly people, or those with heart disease, should take great care if starting this practice and only do so gradually. Gerontologists have noted that many of the long-lived people in Georgia are in the habit of taking a daily dip in often ice-cold pools and streams. This practice gets the blood racing through the body's deeper arteries and causes the more superficial blood vessels to contract vigorously, a process that has been described as 'gymnastics for the arteries'. Most people keep their body surface at a constant, and abnormally high, temperature. By habitually wrapping themselves in a cocoon of warm clothes and sitting in overheated rooms, they keep their skin blood vessels permanently dilated. Fearing the effect of a draught or chill they never expose their bodies to the cold, and so never give their cutaneous arteries a chance to 'flex their muscles' and contract firmly. As a result the blood vessel walls become flabby, and less ready to react should a crisis occur and blood need to be shunted suddenly inwards from the skin to supply the more urgent needs of the brain or heart. This speed of reactivity may be a matter of life or death in cases of post-traumatic shock, heart attack or stroke.

It's been said that a man is as old as his arteries. If so, the Georgian centenarians deserve to retain their juvenile vitality, for in taking their regular cold dips they may have discovered the 'Fountain of Youth'. Studies carried out by Dr A. Fonarev, a Russian biological scientist, show that when the body is exposed to cold water the surface blood vessels contract and so force blood inwards to the heart, brain, intestines, liver and spleen. This can be a boon to the internal organs as well as a way of encouraging a high degree of bodily vigour. But the greatest advantage of 'water fortification', according to the Russian doctor, is that it tunes up the body's thermoregulatory mechanism, so that an equable body temperature can be easily maintained even under the most extreme climactic conditions. Take a daily shower in cold water and you'll quickly lose your fear of wintry weather, and soon find that you look forward with enjoyment to this invigorating early morning stimulus.

If you decide to make this practice part of your dynamogenic routine keep the showers brief, and always end them with a brisk rubdown with a rough Turkish towel, loofah or skin mitten. This will enliven the skin and give you a delicious warm glow from head to toe. A cold bath or shower shouldn't leave you with your teeth chattering and your skin blue. If it does, either you've been exposed to the cold too long, or you're not yet fit enough to take this Spartan therapy. In this case switch to having a tepid shower, and gradually lower the temperature of the water as the reactivity of your circulation improves.

A healthy naturalism should fashion every aspect of our lives, from the way we dress to the way we sleep and eat. Why wear fashion shoes that cripple the feet and make walking uncomfortable? If footwear must be worn, it should be functionally designed and anatomically shaped to fit the feet. The test of a satisfactory pair of shoes is not that it appears to provide a snug fit in the shop, but that it permits you to walk easily, and hop, skip and dance without discomfort. If you can't run a hundred yards in a pair of shoes throw them away, for it's no economy to keep shoes that constrict your feet and cramp your style. Whenever possible dispense with footwear altogether, and walk about unshod. This will allow the toes to expand, and give the foot's complement of thirty-three separate joints some much-needed exercise.

Listen to the wisdom of your body. If your shoes feel like overtight girdles, kick them off. If you're too hot for comfort, shed a layer of clothing. When the pangs of hunger gnaw at your stomach, eat. When you feel satiated, stop. If you feel happy, laugh. Frolic when you feel frisky. Rest when you feel tired. In this way you'll be more closely in tune with your mood, and more likely to meet your body's physiological needs.

In your choice of diet always prefer natural foods to processed foods, and raw foods to cooked foods. The human body was evolved to cope with a Stone Age diet of meat, whole grain cereals, fruit and nuts, not a sophisticated mishmash of chips, cakes, biscuits, synthetic custards, ersatz puddings and ketchup. Stick to natural foods and you'll avoid the risk of side effects from the thousands of chemicals added to modern processed foods. If you make your own oil and vinegar salad dressing you'll avoid the emulsifiers and stabilizers which are used to prepare commercial salad dressing. Bake your own bread and you'll escape the commercial baker's chemical *pot-pourri* of potassium bromate (used to age and strengthen the dough), chlorine dioxide (flour bleach), sodium diacetate (mould inhibitor), glyceryl monostearate (fat extender for making the dough smoother) and nitrogen peroxide (maturing agent needed for short-rise baking process). You'll also have an end product which doesn't taste like shredded blotting paper. Make your own wine and you avoid the chemicals that go into the *vin ordinaires* of some commercial vintners – the azo dye used to supply a richer burgundy colour, the metatartaric acid which inhibits crystal formation, and the heavy doses of sulphuric acid which check bacterial growth. (The World Health Organization recommends a maximum dose of 100 mg of sulphur dioxide a day – a dosage which may be contained in a single half-litre bottle of some cheap white wines.)

Eating raw, natural foods will also increase your intake of vegetable fibre, a vital food factor which the food industry has gone to enormous lengths to remove from our diet. Flour has been milled to remove its fibrous outer casing and produce a whiter, longer lasting loaf. Rice and sugar have been de-husked, and new strains of tomatoes and carrots developed with a reduced fibre content to satisfy consumer demand for soft, pappy foods. As a result of this 'refining' process, it's estimated that during the last ninety years the fibre content of our diet has fallen by a massive 300 per cent. This, it is now realized, has had an insidious effect on our health. Studies have shown that individuals whose diets are deficient in roughage are more prone to develop constipation, diverticulitis, bowel cancer, varicose veins, haemorrhoids, heart disease and obesity, so now we're being advised to sprinkle our denatured soups and breakfast cereals with bran. But a much more satisfactory way of ensuring an adequate intake of vegetable fibre is to revert to eating raw fruits, vegetables and wholemeal bread rather than highly refined convenience foods such as cakes, biscuits, sugar, sweets, ice-cream and white flour products.

People who go on a Stone Age diet find that their energy rises and their weight falls. This is partly because natural foods can never be such rich sources of calories as biscuits, sweets and sugar, and partly because eating concentrated foodstuffs can play havoc with the body's normal appetite-regulating mechanism. Compare, for example, the effects of eating an apple and drinking a glass of apple juice. Tests carried out on a group of volunteers at the Bristol Royal Infirmary show that apple juice is consumed eleven times faster than a whole apple. As it does less to satisfy the appetite, more of the juice is consumed, which means that the total intake of calories is increased. In addition, while eating an apple leads to a relatively slow release of energy, drinking the juice causes a sudden rise of blood sugar. This provokes an increased output of insulin to remove the excess sugar from the circulation, and leads to a rebound plummetting of the blood sugar level. The result is a feeling of hunger and fatigue which then is generally assuaged by further eating.

So the pattern of overeating is established with calorie-rich foods being converted into fat for storage, rather than used as sources of immediate energy. Television commercials may promote the energy-giving potential of chocolate bars and patent breakfast cereals, but for long term energy release there is no substitute for natural foods such as nuts, raisins, apples, potatoes, wholemeal bread and cheese.

Lead an unsophisticated, outdoor life – fresh air, sunlight, sensible clothing to wear and wholesome food to eat – and you'll escape some of the major hazards of urban living.

Dynamogenic step three: Take no drugs unless they are medically essential

While few would question the life-saving value of insulin for a diabetic, or streptomycin and PAS for a sufferer from tuberculosis, there can be no doubt that medicines nowadays are being overprescribed on an enormous scale. According to an estimate made by Professor T. Higuchi, Professor of Pharmaceutical Chemistry at the University of Kansas, approximately nine out of every ten drugs administered today are unnecessary. This practice helps to swell the revenues of the pharmaceutical companies, and would be of little concern if the medicaments were as innocuous as the evil-tasting coloured waters of yesterday. But modern drugs are powerful, and any drug which can be a power for good can equally well be a power for ill if wrongly used. Whole textbooks are being written now on the iatrogenic diseases – the diseases caused as side effects of modern medication. According to Nobel Prize-winner Andrew Lwoff, nearly a third of the illness in France today is caused by the abuse of medically prescribed drugs. Even more alarming is the wholesale misuse of over-the-counter medicaments.

Vast numbers of people lack vitality because they are going about in a permanently drugged state. Consider the side effects of some of the most widely prescribed drugs. The antihistamine medicaments, so profusely administered to relieve colds, insect bites and minor skin irritations, can cause drowsiness – so much so that in Britain bottles of antihistamine pills are forced by law to carry the warning: 'Caution. This may cause drowsiness. If affected do not drive or operate machinery.' (The German Auto Club has published a list of *two hundred* ethical pharmaceutical products that can impair driving performance, and reckons that this list may well swell to include about a thousand drugs when its chemists have had a chance to investigate all the 55,000 drugs available for sale on the German market.) The effects of sleeping pills, which some doctors hand out like winegums, may persist for many hours. If taken last thing at night they can cause feelings of tiredness and apathy which persist well into the following day. Likewise travel sickness pills, tranquillizers and antihypertensive drugs, which can all have a depressant effect on bodily activity.

Other drugs cause fatigue, indirectly, by provoking anaemia and so lowering the oxygen-carrying capacity of the blood. The most common of these is aspirin, which is consumed in America at the rate of 175 tonnes a week, or more than enough to supply every man, woman and child with two tablets a day. This is a common cause of gastrointestinal bleeding, studies having shown that gastric haemorrhages arise in two out of every three people who take the relatively modest dose of three to four aspirin tablets a day.

Most of these pills are taken to suppress pains which should be treated in other ways. Health can't be obtained from a bottle. You may be able to deaden the symptoms of a tension headache with analgesic drugs but you can't relieve the underlying trouble in this way. In the same way, given a sufficiently powerful laxative the most costive bowels can be made to move, but only a modification of diet and a change of dietary habit is likely to cure a case of chronic constipation. This is one of the most tragic consequences of taking patent medicines – it lulls people into a false sense of security and encourages them to settle for a state of sub-health in which the successful suppression of disease symptoms is taken as a sign of physical fitness. But health is a positive state, and not merely the absence of recognizable illness. You'll never be dynamogenically fit if you continue to swallow painkillers, antacids, cold cures, aperients, tranquillizers, slimming pills and sedatives.

The same applies to other toxic chemicals, such as alcohol, tobacco and the exhaust fumes from cars, which can also have a dampening effect on human vitality. When alcohol is taken in moderation there is no doubt that a little bit of what you fancy does you good. When consumed in small quantities it confers the following benefits:

1. It relaxes. Tests have shown that certain tasks can be performed better after taking a glass or two of sherry, because people are less tense. Performance deteriorates the moment they drink more.
2. It fosters social intercourse. A trial at the Boston State Hospital has revealed that a pint of beer can be a more effective therapeutic agent for geriatric patients than thioridazine, a psychotropic drug they are frequently given.
3. It stimulates digestion. Alcohol increases the flow of the gastric juices – a fact known to St Paul who advised his followers to 'use a little wine for thy stomach's sake.'
4. It's bactericidal. Just as surgical spirit is employed to cleanse the skin, so a little wine can be used to kill intestinal germs. Canadian researchers have discovered that wine (particularly red wine) reduces the activity of many of the viral inhabitants of the human intestine.
5. It aids the circulation. Alcohol dilates the peripheral blood vessels and reduces the blood pressure. This makes it a valuable medicine for anyone suffering from narrowing of the arteries or an elevated blood pressure. Alcohol has the additional pharmacological property of lowering the blood cholesterol level and so reducing the risk of arteriosclerosis. This explains why alcoholics are normally found to have remarkably clean, unblocked arteries on post-mortem examination.
6. It prolongs life. Studies of the long-lived communities in Ecuador and the Caucasian mountains show that they invariably enjoy a modest, but regular consumption of alcohol. This is confirmed by American actuarial studies which show that moderate drinkers tend to live longer on average than either heavy drinkers or total abstainers.

Alcohol is, therefore, a wholly acceptable part of the

dynamogenic way of life, *providing* it's not consumed in unreasonable quantities. Take it in excess, however, and it immediately ceases to be a medicine and becomes instead a highly toxic drug.

It's impossible to be full of mental and physical energy if you're under the sedation of large quantities of spirits, beer or wine. In this state your muscles will be slack, your reflexes slowed and your mental processes dulled. (American research work suggests that a few brain cells are killed whenever people drink to the point of feeling slightly giddy, with as many as ten thousand brain cells being destroyed after a heavy drinking spree.) Excessive drinking can also impair your sex life – a fact which is often embarrassingly obvious in men where, in Shakespeare's words, it 'increases the desire but takes away the performance'.

To get the benefits of alcohol without suffering any of its attendant risks, it's necessary to drink in strict moderation. Just over a century ago a Scottish doctor, Dr Francis Anstie, laid down the safety limit for drinkers as 42 ml (1½ fl oz) of alcohol a day. This is equivalent to a daily ration of half a bottle of wine, two pints of beer or three and a half single measures of whisky. Recent research confirms the soundness of this advice. As the US Health Department stated in a recent report *Alcohol and Health*, 'The classical Anstie's Limit seems still to reflect the safe amount of drinking.' But even when this limit is strictly observed, it's advisable to exercise certain additional precautions to avoid suffering the toxic effects of alcohol. These include sipping drinks slowly and never drinking on an empty stomach. Safest of all, perhaps, is the ritual of the gentle sundowner, taken when the day's work is over. This makes a pleasant and relaxing end to the day, and an excellent preparation for a sound night's sleep.

Smoking is a totally different proposition. Moderate drinking has its assets, but there are no redeeming features about the tobacco habit. Everything about this practice is inimicable to the dynamogenic way of life. Here are five of the ways in which smoking reduces vitality and health:

1. It shortens life. Smokers have a one-in-three chance of dying prematurely from lung cancer, bronchitis, emphysema or heart disease.

2. It lowers resistance to infection. Smoking impairs the effectiveness of the body's antibody system and reduces the vitality of the phagocyte cells in the blood, which have the prime responsibility for combating germs. Animal experiments suggest that eighty per cent of this lowered resistance is regained within four months of stopping smoking.

3. It impairs breathing. Smoking irritates the lungs and narrows the bronchial tubes. Tests show that ninety per cent of this lost lung function is regained within nine months of quitting smoking.

4. It decreases vitality. Cigarette smoke contains considerable quantities of carbon monoxide – a poisonous gas which blocks the transmission of oxygen throughout the body by combining with the haemoglobin in the blood to form carboxyhaemoglobin. In this way stamina and vitality are reduced. Tests carried out in anti-smoking clinics in Sweden show that physical fitness improves by as much as twenty per cent within a month of giving up smoking.

5. It impairs sexual performance. Tobacco advertisements try to suggest that smoking enhances a man's vigour, potency and sex appeal. But there's nothing appealing about catarrh, bad breath, stained fingers and a hacking cough. Recent research has also shown that smoking can lower male fertility by reducing sperm mobility, and there is clinical evidence that smoking can also hamper sexual enjoyment, possibly by decreasing the output of testosterone, the male sex hormone. As Dr Alton Ochsner, head of a famous American anti-smoking clinic, has observed, 'Many men don't recognize that

they have a libido problem until after they have stopped smoking and then they realize what they've been missing.'

In view of this incriminatory evidence, no one who wants to lead a long, vigorous and healthy life should smoke. Nor should they spend too long inhaling polluted city air, for car engines are another common source of carbon monoxide. Every year in Britain cars belch out somewhere in the region of five million tons of carbon monoxide gas. Most of this toxic gas escapes harmlessly into the atmosphere, but in crowded city streets the carbon monoxide levels sometimes exceed the maximum safety limits permitted in industry. This can make people feel tired, dizzy and slightly nauseous. Within the interior of cars idling in city traffic jams the concentration of carbon monoxide can be higher still. In fact, one doctor who has made a special study of the subject claims that, 'In any street most people in cars are in a partly drugged state.' To avoid this hazard make a point of switching off your car engine as quickly as possible in confined spaces such as garages, underground car parks and car ferries; check that your exhaust system is in good repair and not leaking fumes into the passenger compartment; switch off your air intake in dense, slowly moving traffic to avoid sucking in fumes from the car in front (engines generate four times as much carbon monoxide when they're driven at normal cruising speeds); and keep your car properly serviced, since dirty sparking plugs and badly adjusted carburettors can double the output of carbon monoxide. Better still, keep away from fume-filled city streets, and enjoy whenever possible the exhilaration of the fresh country air.

You'll never be brimming over with vitality if your body is saturated with drugs.

Dynamogenic step four: Live passionately
Civilization has placed a curb on both our physical and affective lives. The construction of machines has given us

less chance to give vent to our physical energy, and the creation of strict social conventions and taboos has severely curtailed our release of emotional energy. As a result, our lives have become increasingly unexciting, passive and routine.

Freud, in his seminal work *Civilization and its Discontents*, claimed that there was an irremediable conflict between the instinctual needs of the individual, and the demands of polite society. The whole framework of our closely knit communities would be threatened if we were free to make spontaneous expression of our instinctual feelings and obtain immediate gratification of our animal lusts. We cannot grab the apples from a farmer's orchard to assuage our hunger, or urinate in the street whenever our bladders are uncomfortably full. Nor can we punch the paper boy on the nose simply because we can't abide his off-key whistling, or fornicate at will with our neighbours just because they are sexually appealing and happen to be passing by. We must accept some social restraints if we are going to live in communal harmony. But need we maintain such a tight rein on our emotions?

At school we are taught to keep a cool head so that we can make dispassionate judgements. We're told that rational decisions can't be made in a state of high emotion. So we learn to exclude all feelings from our intellectual deliberations and debates. But modern men and women are thinking animals and spend a large part of their day in rational thought, analysing the past, puzzling about the present, and attempting to predict the future. As a result we spend an increasing part of our lives keeping a tight rein on our emotions, and holding back the spontaneous expression of 'irrational' feelings. We think more, but feel less.

In infancy we are trained to repress our instinctual needs. In childhood we are taught to exclude all feelings that might hamper our faculty for cold calculation. Later on in life we discover that we can shield ourselves from the slings and arrows of outrageous fortune by building an impregnable screen around our emotions. In this way we feel no pain, but neither can we feel any pleasure. Psychologist Rollo May sees this schizoid withdrawal as the sickness of the age. Our prevailing mood is one of cold aloofness. Depending on our generation we're either 'laid back', 'playing it cool' or 'keeping a stiff upper lip'. We are apathetic in the true meaning of the word, because we are *a-pathos* – without feeling.

This culturally contrived state of emotional anaesthesia is anathema to the dynamogenic way of life. You can't be either healthy, happy or successful if you place a bar on your emotional life. As philosopher Bertrand Russell said, 'Zest is the secret of happiness and well-being.' To extract from each day the fullest measure of excitement and joy you've got to plunge headlong into the maelstrom of life. If you want a thoroughly fulfilling sex life you must abandon your childhood inhibitions and revel unashamedly in the exciting exchanges of mutual love. If you want to share the gourmet's delight in eating you must first cultivate the gourmet's all-absorbing interest in food, its careful preparation, mouth-watering appearance, and delicate flavour. If you want to develop a wide circle of close and rewarding friendships, you yourself must be warm, caring and passionately interested in people, for what we receive from social relationships is in direct proportion to what we bring to them. Fulfilment comes from commitment, in both friendship and love.

This total emotional commitment is also the pathway to success. As Ralph Waldo Emerson observed, 'Nothing great was ever achieved without enthusiasm.' What would Joan of Arc, a simple girl from Orleans, have accomplished had she not been inspired by religious zeal? Would Columbus have discovered the West Indies and America had he not been driven by a fervent desire to find a Western passageway to the Orient? The history of the world is the story of dedicated men and women like these – people whose passionate interests and desires have motivated them to overcome frustration, ridicule,

259

failure, poverty and sickness in the single-minded pursuit of their goals. Faced with this boundless energy and enthusiasm, impossibilities vanish.

But how do we overcome the restraints imposed by our emotionally repressive upbringing and unleash the motive power of our instinctual drive? How do we recapture the freedom and joy of honest, spontaneous emotional expression? Only by patient behavioural retraining. We must learn to let ourselves go and be more spontaneous (see page 74). We must be prepared to take more risks (see page 180). And we must strive to get in closer touch with our bodies, for these are sounding boards for the emotions. The affections of love, fear and anger would be pale, emaciated states were it not for the bodily changes which accompany them. Who can envisage love without the moist eyes, pounding heart and sighing breath? Or contemplate anger unaccompanied by a red face, flashing eyes, and tense, trembling body? If we attempt to suppress these physiological changes we kill the emotions which give them birth. Instead of putting a damper on our feelings we ought to allow them to resonate throughout our entire bodies, and thrill us to the core. In this way we will know more clearly what is going on in the deep recesses of our brain. So too will our loved ones and friends, who will find it easier to understand us and to respond to our changing moods and unspoken needs.

We must also rediscover the long lost art of play, which is just as important for adults as it is for children. In moments of play we have a chance to express our feelings and let off steam in a socially acceptable way. At these times we break free from the rigid framework of our normal routine lives, and gain the opportunity of exploring and testing our new patterns of behaviour. During these precious moments we rediscover that life is fun, and not the dreadfully serious tragedy that the media constantly portray. In play we lift our spirits, ease our tensions and forge closer relationships with our friends. It is an important character-moulding activity. This was shown when psychiatrist Erik Erikson investigated the personalities of a large group of people, first when they were children, and then thirty years later when they had matured. At this later stage he found that the adults leading the most interesting, fulfilling lives were the ones who had managed to keep a sense of playfulness at the centre of their lives. This bears out the judgement of Plato who, when asked what is the right way of living, replied, 'Life must be lived as play.'

People who lead abundant emotional lives invariably have a catholicity of interests. They benefit by having a well-balanced diet of activities, enlivened by the spice of regular change. Routine, however cosy it may be to begin with, always palls if pursued too long. Human experience is like a kaleidoscope. If you're bored with the current scene, tip your life upside down, give it a vigorous shake, and another pattern will emerge.

Variety of occupation helps to preserve mental health, not only by avoiding boredom, but also by preventing healthy passions from becoming obsessive manias. It is excellent to enjoy good eating, savour excellent wine and revel in the thrills of risk-taking, but disastrous to develop any one of these interests to the point of becoming a glutton, dipsomaniac or compulsive gambler.

Dynamogenic individuals are characterized by their spontaneity, playfulness, widespread interests and insatiable curiosity. Throughout their lives they retain a passionate inquisitiveness about all that is happening around them. They are always avid for new experiences, constantly anxious to explore, discover, understand and learn. Their personalities are not fossilized, but constantly growing. They are always open to novelty and change. Martha Graham, one of the pioneers of modern dance, was just such a person. Throughout her long and distinguished career she kept a close eye on the passing scene and was constantly experimenting with new dance forms. During her lifetime she created over 150 dance dramas and contributed more works to the theatre than any other woman. She was motivated by a passion for life and a zest for new experiences which never deserted her. When interviewed at the age of eighty-two, and asked for the secret of her vitality and creative drive, she said, 'I am hungry, avid for every sensation I can get.' People with that attitude never grow old, nor do their lives grow stale.

Physical activity is a great spur to bodily metabolism, but so too is emotional activity. When we are emotionally excited, physiological changes arise in our body which are identical to those which occur when we indulge in strenuous exercise. When we fall in love or stand on a soap box and preach passionately against the cruelty inflicted on battery-reared animals, our blood pressure soars, our pulse rate rises and our breathing deepens just as if we were running up a flight of stairs. We recognize this in our everyday speech, when we describe these emotive moments when our hearts pound and our breath comes in short pants. Conversely, if we achieve emotional disengagement from the world our metabolism slows. During periods of meditation oxygen consumption falls, the heartbeat slows, and the brain becomes becalmed. This may be a valuable skill to acquire and practise occasionally, but it is no way to achieve a long, productive, vital life.

To achieve our full potential we need to lead lives which are both motive and emotive. Energy and passion need to be in joint harness if we are to attain the full limits of our dynamogenic powers.

Dynamogenic step five: Establish the habit of deep relaxed breathing
Each year millions of pounds are spent on pick-me-ups, nerve foods, tonic wines and vitamin pills. Most of these panaceas are expensive, some are potentially harmful, but none serve the purpose for which they are intended. Pharmacologists dispute the whole idea of general pur-

pose medicinal tonics. If people are anaemic they may need iron pills, but only after the cause of their iron deficiency anaemia has been established. If they are chronically tired, the rational approach is to find, and remedy, the cause of their unnatural fatigue, not to temporarily suppress their unhealthy symptoms with strychnine-based restoratives – a palliative procedure which is no more effective than whipping a tired horse.

Chemical tonics of this kind have no place in modern medical practice. But that is not to decry all pick-me-up remedies. There is one natural elixir which the body constantly and urgently requires, and that is oxygen. This is the very fuel of life – the vital element without which our cells would die in a matter of minutes. Yet when people set out to enliven the function of their weary bodies they will feed them at great expense with glycerophosphates, yeast, glucose and black strap molasses, but rarely think to provide them with a richer supply of oxygen, the most essential nourishment of all. Possibly this is because oxygen is too commonplace to warrant their attention. They can envisage their bodies going short of a comparatively scarce substance like Vitamin E, but with the earth's atmosphere one-fifth full of oxygen, they cannot possibly imagine that their systems could suffer from hypoxaemia. But it is only by breathing properly that we can ensure the optimum functioning of our heart, brain, kidneys, hormonal glands, muscles and liver. In a world of plenty, it is possible for us to be suffering our own internal energy crisis.

This prophylactic fact was better appreciated by our forebears than it is today. They had little idea of respiratory physiology, but realized that breathing was essential for the maintenance of health. To them it was primarily a way of absorbing the mysterious life force which animated the natural world. The ancient Hebrews spoke of the 'breath of life'. Long before Priestley discovered oxygen, yogis strove to control the intake of *prana*, the vital force contained in the air which, they

263

recognized, gave animation to both body and mind. The Romans shared the same belief and used the single word *spiritus* to describe both 'breath' and 'life force', and it is from this common root that we derive such words as *spirited* and *inspiration*, which describe the states of exuberant physical energy and mental creativity which arise when we are enthused by the respiratory life force.

If you want a bodily tonic or mental stimulant you can do no better than increase your intake of oxygen. As Voltaire said two hundred years ago, 'A good deal of human illness could be cured by breathing.'

This particularly applies today when people spend so much of their time indoors in polluted atmospheres, and lead such inactive lives that their lungs are rarely brought into full play. The tension of modern life also accentuates the tendency to shallow breathing. When we are anxious our breathing tends to come in short, nervous pants. If continued too long this pattern of breathing can give rise to a condition known medically as The Hyperventilation Syndrome. Under normal conditions we breathe about 16 to 18 times a minute. When under stress this rate can increase to 22 or more. The main effect of this nervous over-breathing is to increase the amount of carbon dioxide voided from the body. This alters the chemistry of the blood and produces symptoms of anxiety – rapid pulse rate, numbness, pins and needles of the hands and feet, faintness and a tendency to cramp. In this way an initial feeling of mild anxiety can be converted into a full-blown panic state. The long-term solution to this problem is to cultivate a deeper, more relaxed pattern of breathing (A quicker remedy is to hold the breath for a few seconds, which will retain carbon dioxide in the lungs long enough to restore the normal chemistry of the blood.)

People who inhibit the free expression of their feelings are also likely to become tense, shallow breathers. Most emotional states are associated with a change in our pattern of respiration. When we're bored we yawn, when we're startled we catch our breath, when we're surprised we gasp, and when we're suffering from unrequited love we sigh like a furnace. If we want to suppress our awareness of our emotional state, or hide our feelings from others, these respiratory changes need to be checked. This is a further reason for restricted breathing, and according to Reichean therapists, a common cause of psychosomatic illness. As Wilhelm Reich himself observed, 'it has become clear that the inhibition of respiration was the physiological mechanism for the suppression and repression of emotion, and consequently the basic mechanism of neurosis.' Various methods have been devised to overcome these inhibiting tensions. Some therapists encourage their patients to cry, others to give vent to their repressed screams, or to indulge in uninhibited laughter. But screaming, laughter and crying are merely modified forms of breathing. Their only therapeutic value is that they allow people to overcome their respiratory tensions and so restore a natural pattern of breathing. In this way they escape the burden of their inhibitions and neurotic anxieties by literally getting them off their chest.

Dynamogenic living needs the support of dynamogenic breathing. The lungs consist of a mass of approximately 300 million tiny air sacs, or *alveoli*, linked together like two enormous bunches of grapes. Together they form an expanse more than forty times the surface area of the body. Around each air sac is a network of delicate blood vessels, which are just wide enough to allow the red blood corpuscles to circulate in single file. Each corpuscle remains in contact with the aveolar wall for about three-quarters of a second, during which time it has to discharge its content of carbon dioxide waste, and replenish its store of oxygen. The conscious practice of deep breathing enhances this vital exchange, by promoting the uptake of oxygen and facilitating the elimination of carbon dioxide waste. It also aids the elimination of many other waste products from the body, for the lungs are as much organs of excretion as the kidneys. This fact is often overlooked, unless you happen to be a frequent passenger of the Paris Metro and smell the garlic-laden air. But research has shown that the lungs play an important part in ridding the body of excess quantities of histamine, serotonin and alcohol. (Hence the breathalysing of drivers to determine the amount of alcohol they have consumed.)

To establish the habit of correct breathing, adopt the following three principles:

1. Always breathe through the nose. The nasal passages, with their complicated system of convoluted bones and cartilages, provide a highly efficient air-conditioning system. Experiments with animals have shown that the nose can process dirty air at temperatures ranging from as high as 500°C (932°F) to as low as −100°C and pass it on to the lungs cleaned and warmed to approximately body temperature. It's estimated that during an average day we inhale 20,000 million particles of dirt and dust. Providing the air is taken in through the nose and not through the mouth, all these particles are trapped by the sticky film of mucus which covers the nasal passages and then wafted out of harm's way by millions of fine hairs, or *cilia*.

Another advantage of breathing through the nose is that it helps to clear the sinuses. The drainage of these cavities was no problem when man walked about on all four limbs. Now that we have assumed the upright position, the cavity and bases of some of our sinuses have come to lie below their openings. This means they can no longer be drained by gravity alone, but require a suction force to expel their contents. This is created, as it is in an aerosol paint spray, whenever a strong current of air is drawn across the openings of the sinuses. As a result, habitual mouth-breathers are considerably more likely to suffer congested sinuses and catarrh than those who always breathe through the nose. Since they bypass their natural germ filter, they're also more prone to develop sore throats and chest infections. But more important still, by breathing unwarmed air they bring about a reflex contraction of their bronchial tubes which can substantially reduce the volume of oxygen they inspire.

2. Breathe deeply. A sedentary worker uses only a small fraction of his total lung capacity. People who adopt the dynamogenic programme, and get their full quota of activity units a week, automatically give their lungs a fuller airing. When they're running, swimming, skipping or dancing they ventilate the little-used areas at the apex and base of the lungs, increase the lungs' vital capacity and raise the rate of oxygen uptake from the alveoli. But this doesn't necessarily maintain an optimum intake of oxygen during the rest of their lives. During the times when they're not exercising they can still revert to their old pattern of shallow breathing. This fault can be overcome by making a practice of breathing deeply at regular periods during the day. During the night our respiration sinks to the lowest possible maintenance level. As a result we tend to feel drowsy when we wake and instinctively yawn to take in one or two extra gulps of air. This arousal process can be assisted by performing just one minute's deep breathing immediately after getting out of bed, preferably in front of an open window. This is all that's necessary to recharge your blood with oxygen and get your morning off to a flying start. (Taking an early morning cold shower will have the same effect.)

If during the day you feel in need of a quick energy boost, don't grab a cigarette or swallow a quick cup of coffee, but take instead a few refreshing draughts of air. This will quickly perk you up and restore your flagging energy. Every time you read a paper or journal make a point of filling your lungs and reading the occasional paragraph on just a single breath. And when you walk, establish the routine of breathing in for the count of five steps to fill the lungs to the full, then out again for the following six strides until the last particle of air has been driven from your lungs. Incidentally, you may find if you do the deep breathing routine too rapidly that you go light-headed after a few deep breaths. If so, breathe normally for a while and it will pass.

Another possible benefit of deep breathing is that it can help to keep you slim. This is one of the major weight-reducing measures employed by Dr Lothar G. Tirala, head of the eminent Walke Sanatorium in Wiesbaden, Germany. He has found that many overweight people breathe badly and can be helped to regain a normal weight balance without the need for fasting and starvation regimes simply by placing them on a balanced diet supplemented by deep breathing exercises. The rationale of this approach is easy to follow. By taking deep breaths the intake of oxygen is increased. This acts as the bellows which fan the body's metabolic fires, and so steps up the rate at which fat is consumed.

(When performing these lung-expanding exercises, remember the tip of briefly holding the breath at the point of maximum inhalation, which lengthens the time the freshly-inspired air is kept in contact with the alveoli, and can increase the oxygenation of the blood by as much as 25 per cent.)

3. Exhale fully. You can't fill a bottle with fresh water until you first empty out its contents of stale liquid. In the same way it's impossible to replenish the lungs with a new supply of oxygen-rich air while they're still saturated with devitalized air. A large part of the secret of healthy breathing is therefore to ensure the adequate emptying of the lungs. Even when we breathe to the maximum of our ability only one sixth of the air in the lungs gets changed, a fraction that is considerably reduced with a more shallow tidal air change. Breathe out to the full and you'll ensure the easy intake of a deep, revivifying draught of air.

Deep expiration is also an aid to relaxation. When we're in a stressful situation we take an involuntary inward gasp and prepare ourselves for action by tensing the muscles of our abdomen and chest. When the danger is over we give a sigh of relief and automatically relax from head to toe. By consciously controlling our breathing we can exercise a considerable measure of control over these tension states. If you have an after-dinner speech to give and can feel your pulse racing, and the muscles in your throat knotting up, control your mounting anxiety by consciously regulating your breathing. For a few moments make a point of breathing slowly, deeply and rhythmically. Concentrate in particular on breathing out. Imagine that you're a hot air balloon collapsing slowly to the ground. This will dispel your tension like ice melting in the full glare of the summer sun. Follow the yoga practice of focusing your attention on the passage of air in and out of your nostrils. Feel your nostrils flare as you breathe in and out and compare the coolness of the air you inhale with the gentle warmth of the air which leaves your lungs. If you find this sensation difficult to appreciate, concentrate instead on intoning the word 'calm' as you expire. By focusing your attention in this way you'll take your mind off worrying thoughts, and by exhaling deeply and rhythmically you'll coax your body into a state of profound relaxation.

The same mental imagery can be employed when you take your daily constitutional. When you breathe in repeat to yourself the words 'Life ... life ... life' with every step you take. This will make you more fully aware of the fact that as you inspire you are absorbing oxygen, the life force. Then when you breathe out silently chant the words 'Peace ... peace ... peace' to maximize the relaxation of your body. In this way you will acquire the hallmark of all healthy animals – the ability to swing rapidly from a state of quiet repose to one of vigorous action.

Dynamogenic step six: Observe the Reveille Ritual every morning
One of the penalties of sedentary living is that it fosters

stiffness. Keeping the body supple was no problem when man's life entailed clambering into caves, stalking wild animals, and climbing trees for nuts and fruits. Varied activities like these automatically kept the body lissom. Not so today. Now there is little need to bend, stretch and twist. Everything nowadays is devised to spare the need for movement. Shoe horns are constructed with long handles, cookers set at eye-level height and stairs made with a rise rarely more than seven inches in height. As a result of this calculated policy of unemployment our joints stiffen, our ligaments shorten and our muscles contract. This makes our movements ungainly, stiff and cumbersome. In time it becomes difficult even to carry out such simple actions as getting out of a chair or bending down to fasten a pair of shoes. However young we happen to be this gives us the stamp of premature senility, for stiffness is synonymous with old age, and is the characteristic mimicked by actors whenever they want to play the part of an elderly person.

Rigidity also detracts from physical attraction, which depends not only on beauty of figure and face, but also on grace of carriage and ease and elegance of movement. People who are stiff are also more prone to injury and rheumatic disease (see page 92). To maintain the health of our joints we need to put them through their entire range of movements at least once a day. But how often does the average person fully utilize his hips? How often, for example, do we flex our knees to touch our chest? Unless we're contortionists, ballet dancers or keep-fit instructors, the chances are that we don't perform this movement once a month, let alone once a day. As a result, our hip joints suffer the degeneration of disuse, and become prone to osteoarthritic changes. Orthopaedic surgeons now offer a wonderful replacement service for decayed hip joints, but they are no substitute for the real thing. If you keep your joints supple you'll have no need for crutches, spinal jackets and spare part surgery.

Many people believe that bowed bodies and stiff joints

are an inevitable accompaniment of the ageing process. But this is not true. I have had patients who have maintained an upright carriage and an excellent flexibility of movement well into their nineties by having regular osteopathic treatment to maintain the suppleness of their joints. I have also had patients who once needed regular manipulative treatment for their stiff necks and aching backs but have overcome these recurrent problems by taking up yoga. When I've had the opportunity to examine them at a later date I have found them more supple at seventy than they were in their fifties and sixties. This proves that increasing stiffness is the retribution of neglect, not the penalty of age. Keep yourself supple and you can retain a graceful, upright posture and a youthful flexibility and ease of movement well into your eighties and even nineties.

Instead of sparing yourself the need for physical contortions during the day, go out of your way whenever possible to bend and stretch your joints. Before you go to sleep at night hug your knees to your chest in the extreme foetal position. This will stretch out the lower part of your back and get rid of some of the spinal tensions that have accumulated during the day. When you wake up in the morning loosen your neck by rolling your head from side to side on the pillow. Put the joints of your ankles and feet through their paces by turning a complete circle with each foot whenever you put on your socks and shoes or tights. When you dry your back after a bath or shower take the opportunity to exercise your shoulder joints by grasping the towel behind you and gently coaxing each hand to travel as far as possible up and down your back. When you climb the stairs, don't be content to go up step by step, but give your hip joints a more thorough stretch by spanning two or three steps at a time. On country walks clamber over stiles rather than walking through gates, and in the evenings dispense occasionally with chairs and rest instead on cushions on the floor. In this way you'll escape the postural strain of sitting and also put your body through a wide range of mobilizing exercises when you shift your position and ring the changes between lying prone, reclining on the side, squatting on the haunches and sitting cross-legged. If you make bending and stretching a part of your daily routine you'll find it easier to retain a graceful carriage and youthful agility.

But this alone may not be sufficient to keep all your joints in good working order. Despite reaching up to open cupboards and stooping down to make the bed you may still lack the right movement to loosen your shoulders and flex your hips. For this reason it's advisable to follow the example of cats and dogs and start the day by performing a brief series of limbering exercises. These needn't take long, but should be planned in such a way that they maintain the flexibility of the body's major joints, particularly those of the knees, hips, shoulders, back and neck. The following regime – called the Reveille Ritual since it's intended for use first thing in the morning – is designed specifically to meet these needs. It also encourages the upright carriage of the body and improves balance – two attributes that are commonly lost by default with the passage of time. In performing the Reveille Ritual you'll also improve your breathing by increasing the flexibility of the rib cage, which is particularly important for people who slouch over desks, are habitual shallow breathers, or suffer from asthma, chronic bronchitis or emphysema.

Ideally these exercises should be performed in the nude, preferably first thing in the morning, although later in the day is satisfactory providing you're not too tired to do them justice. They should be done slowly, with no attempt at strain. Since the object of the routine is to maintain the full excursion of the joints, it's the last few degrees of every movement that do the most good. So it's more effective to perform one thorough stretch than a score or more of half-hearted stretches. Once you have learned the routine, it should take no more than two or three minutes to execute, since it occupies no longer than the time required to take ten to twelve deep breaths. The only equipment you require is a rod approximately 45 cm (18 in) long which should be kept handy in bedroom or bathroom. A short section of broom handle is ideal for the purpose. Paint this in eye-catching candy stripes and it will act as a permanent reminder to you to carry out your early morning stretching.

Reveille Ritual

1. Stand erect, feet hip width apart, arms relaxed, holding the rod by its ends in front of you with knuckles facing forward.
2. Take a slow, deep breath, and while doing so raise the rod as high as possible over your head, stretching your entire spine upwards as if you were trying to make your head touch the ceiling.
3. When your lungs are fully inflated slowly bend your trunk to the right, exhaling as you go. Make sure when performing this movement that you do not bend forwards and that you keep your head between your arms. At the point of fullest stretch give two or three gentle bounces to coax the spine to bend a little further still. When making these final springing motions shift your pelvis as far as possible to the left, and expel the last few molecules of air from your lungs in a series of audible grunts.
4. When your lungs are fully deflated, slowly return to the upright position with arms raised above your head. Breathe inwards as you go and again stretch as high as possible towards the ceiling.
5. Once the lungs are completely recharged with air slowly repeat the movement to the left. Breathe outwards as you go, and again try to achieve the greatest possible stretching of the spine and hip joint.
6. When full exhalation has been achieved, slowly breathe in and return to the upright, stretching position.
7. After a full breath has been taken, carefully drop the

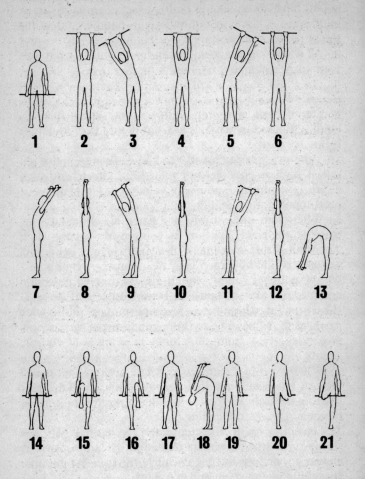

1   2   3   4   5   6

7   8   9   10   11   12   13

14   15   16   17   18   19   20   21

head backwards, breathe out slowly and as you do so bend the spine backwards to its full extent. Once more execute a few gentle bounces at the end point of spinal extension, both to extend the range of movement and to void as much air as possible from the lungs. (Allow the knees to bend naturally during this movement.)

8. As you breathe in return to the erect position and give your neck, spine and rib cage a further upward stretch.

9. Once the point of full inspiration has been reached slowly twist your head and trunk to the right, exhaling as you go. Again execute a series of gentle thrusts to emphasize the final stretch and rotation of the pelvis and spine.

10. When every particle of air has been expelled from your lungs return to the erect position. Slowly replenish your lungs with air and when you've reached the point of maximum inspiration give another upward stretch.

11. Repeat the same sequence turning to the left, breathing out.

12. Return to the erect position and take another full breath in and stretch upward.

13. Now, without applying any force, let the head and trunk sag forwards, allowing the weight of the body to do the work. Exhale slowly, and when you reach the point of furthest flexion perform a few extra bounces to coax the rod towards the ground.

14. When the last particle of air has been driven from your lungs begin to breathe in and slowly return to the starting position, only this time do not raise your arms above your head but leave them hanging limply in front of you.

15. Breathing freely and naturally, balance on your left leg and slowly raise your right leg until your knee is as close as possible to your chest. Thread your right foot through the rod and return it to the ground. (If your balance is poor, and you feel in danger of falling over while doing this, take the precaution of standing in the corner of the room where you have the support, if

needed, of walls on either side.)

16. Repeat the above movement with the other foot, so that the rod is now held behind your back.

17. Hold this position for a few seconds while you take another deep breath.

18. Now exhale slowly and bend the trunk forward, raising the rod as high as possible behind your back while at the same time trying to place your forehead on your knees. Again execute a few bounces and exhalatory grunts to empty the lungs and coax the last few degrees of spinal flexion.

19. Slowly inhale and return to the erect position, with arms hanging loosely behind your back.

20. Breathing freely, balance on your right leg, then bend the left knee and lift it as close as possible to your chest. From this position thread the left knee back through the rod and return it to the ground.

21. Repeat the same movement with the other leg, and return to the upright position.

This completes the sequence of Reveille Ritual, which takes some paragraphs to explain but only a few moments to perform. Repeat this simple routine every day of your life, preferably after an early morning shower, and you'll keep your hips, knees, spine and rib cage in tip-top working order.

Dynamogenic step seven: Three times a week perform the S.H.A.P.E. schedule of exercises

Physical exercise serves three main purposes. In the first place, it increases stamina and improves the performance of the heart and lungs, a function covered in the first step of the dynamogenic programme. The second purpose is to maintain the suppleness of the body, a function achieved by performing the daily Reveille Ritual. The third purpose – maintaining muscular strength – still remains to be considered. People who adopt the dynamogenic way of life will inevitably keep their muscles in better tone than ever before. But it's still

SEMI SQUATS

HEEL RAISE

possible that they may retain a little flabbiness of their tummies and thighs, particularly if they have led a largely sedentary life for many years. To counteract this tendency it's advisable to perform a regular set of muscle-toning exercises. These should concentrate on strengthening the muscles of the legs, arms, chest, abdomen and back. The following schedule is designed for this express purpose. It should be performed three times a week at regular intervals, preferably immediately after carrying out the limbering movements of the Reveille Ritual. (If you have any doubts about your ability to perform this exercise schedule, or suffer from high blood pressure, heart disease or uncontrolled diabetes, consult a doctor before you embark on the routine.)

S.H.A.P.E. Routine
This consists of five basic exercises:

> Semi-squats
> Heel raise
> Abdominal lift
> Press-ups
> Extensor curl.

SEMI-SQUATS Stand erect with hands on hips and feet firmly planted on the ground. Bend the knees until the thighs are parallel with the ground, then immediately straighten the legs and return to the erect position. Repeat this movement ten times in rapid succession. Each week increase the number of semi-squats by two until you are performing a maximum of twenty. Breathe naturally throughout the exercise. (Take care not to sink into a deep knee bend, which can overstretch the knee's supporting ligaments.)

This exercise will strengthen the powerful muscles of the thighs, and make it easier for you to climb hills and run up and down stairs.

HEEL RAISE Stand erect with hands placed on hips. Rise up on the toes as high as you can and then return the

ABDOMINAL LIFT

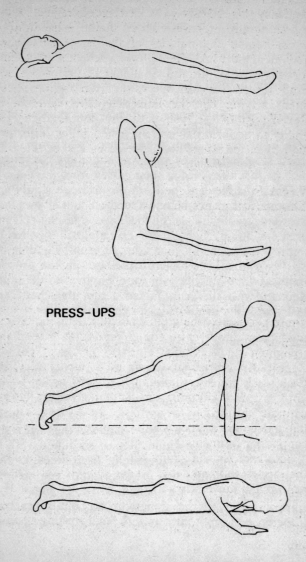

PRESS-UPS

heels to the ground. Repeat ten times in rapid succession. Each week increase the number of rises by two until you are performing a maximum of twenty. Breathe naturally throughout the exercise. This exercise will strengthen the calf muscles and put extra power in your stride.

ABDOMINAL LIFT Lie flat on your back with your hands clasped behind your neck. Slowly raise your trunk until you are in the sitting position, then equally slowly return to the starting position. To begin with perform this exercise only four times, but as your muscles grow stronger slowly increase the number of lifts by two per week until you are doing the exercise a maximum of ten times. If necessary tuck your feet under any convenient piece of furniture to stop them lifting from the floor. If you find it difficult to perform this exercise slowly and smoothly with hands behind your neck and elbows fully extended, try it with arms folded across the chest. If this proves a strain, lighten the exercise still further by keeping your arms by your sides, or even by adding the assistance of a little fingertip pressure on the ground. Then, as your muscles gain tone, progress to doing the exercises with the arms folded across the chest, and finally with the hands clasped behind the neck.

This exercise will improve your posture and give you a firm, flat tummy.

PRESS-UPS Lie face down with body raised from the ground and supported by the hands and toes, with your arms, legs and trunk completely straight. Slowly bend the arms until the chest and forehead lightly touch the ground. Then immediately straighten the arms and resume the starting position. Repeat six times, with no bending of either legs or trunk. Each week as you progress add another two press-ups until you are performing the exercise a maximum of twelve times. If to begin with you lack the strength to carry out this exercise properly, perform it initially with hands resting against a

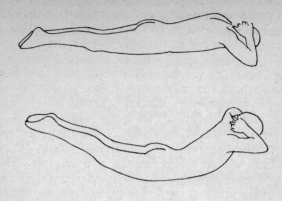

table, and as your muscles gain tone progress to doing it with hands placed on a chair, and finally on the floor.

This exercise will strengthen the muscles of your shoulders and arms, and give you a well-developed chest or firm bustline.

EXTENSOR CURL Lie face down with hands clasped behind your neck. Keeping the legs straight, raise both legs, head and trunk as far as possible from the floor. Hold this position for a few seconds, then return to the starting position. Repeat six times, endeavouring each time to achieve a more extreme hollowing of the back. If the exercise proves difficult to achieve in this form, place your arms straight in front of you and make a start by raising the left arm and the straight right leg as high as possible from the ground. Hold this position briefly, then return to the starting position and raise the opposite arm and leg. This will gradually strengthen your back and enable you to tackle the tougher exercise. Regular

281

performance of this movement will strengthen the important extensor muscles of the back, minimizing the risk of spinal strain and checking any tendency towards round shoulders.

These then are the seven essential steps of dynamogenic living:

Step one: Take a minimum of ten activity units a week;
Step two: Lead a more natural life;
Step three: Take no drugs unless they are medically necessary;
Step four: Live passionately;
Step five: Establish the habit of deep, relaxed breathing;
Step six: Observe the Reveille Ritual every morning;
Step seven: Perform the S.H.A.P.E. schedule of exercises three times a week.

Incorporate these seven principles into your daily life and you'll escape the penalties of hypokinetic living, and gain increased vitality, excitement, sexual vigour and a longer, more productive life.

The Greeks took as their therapeutic aim the establishment of a healthy mind in a healthy body. But they didn't offer a straightforward explanation of how this end could be achieved. Dynamogenics adopts the identical target, and also provides a clear, step-by-step programme through which this goal can be attained. The over-riding motto of the programme, not far removed from that of the Greeks themselves, is 'Mens sana in corpore sano' – a healthy mind in a healthy body. In that single principle lies the secret of human health, happiness and success.

INDEX